Sign or Symptom?

AF737783

Edited by
Tine Van Osselaer
Henk de Smaele
Kaat Wils

SIGN *or* SYMPTOM?

Exceptional Corporeal Phenomena in Religion and Medicine in the Nineteenth and Twentieth Centuries

Leuven University Press

This book appears in the peer-reviewed series
KADOC Studies on Religion, Culture & Society

EDITORIAL BOARD

Urs Altermatt, Université de Fribourg
Timothy Brittain-Catlin, University of Kent
Wilhelm Damberg, Ruhr-Universität Bochum
Jan De Maeyer, KU Leuven - KADOC
Jean-Dominique Durand, Université Lyon 3
Emmanuel Gerard, KU Leuven - KADOC
James C. Kennedy, University College Utrecht
Rupert Klieber, Universität Wien
Mathijs Lamberigts, KU Leuven
Emiel Lamberts, KU Leuven
Jean-Michel Leniaud, École pratique des hautes études, Sorbonne, Paris
Daniele Menozzi, Scuola Normale Superiore di Pisa
Anne Morelli, Université Libre de Bruxelles
Silvia Mostaccio, Université catholique de Louvain
Patrick Pasture, KU Leuven
Liliane Voyé, Université Catholique de Louvain

© 2017 Leuven University Press/Presses universitaires de Louvain/Universitaire Pers Leuven,
Minderbroedersstraat 4, B-3000 Leuven (Belgium)

All rights reserved. Except in those cases expressly determined by law, no part of this publication may be multiplied, saved in an automated data file or made public in any way whatsoever without the express prior written consent of the publishers.

ISBN 978 94 6270 107 6
D/2017/1869/23
NUR: 694

GPRC
Guaranteed
Peer Reviewed
Content
www.gprc.be

CONTENTS

INTRODUCTION

TINE VAN OSSELAER*

Pierre's bones

On 24 May 1899 at five o'clock in the morning, Edouard Duclos and Albin Roels were standing over a grave in the cemetery of Jabbeke, a small village in Flanders. The carpenter and grave digger quickly set to work and, after a short time, they had exhumed a coffin buried only fourteen months earlier. After transporting the remains to the garden of the pastor, Pierre De Vaere, the three men watched Dr Van Hoestenberghe (from Stalhille) inspect the corpse and then amputate both legs just beneath the knee. After removing the feet and as much tissue as possible, Van Hoestenberghe asked the men to close the coffin, taking the legs with him. By seven o'clock, the coffin had been reburied and peace in the cemetery was restored.[1]

Why resort to such extreme measures as exhumation and amputation? Anyone who had inquired after the identity of the corpse that early morning would have had their answer to the question on hearing the name of the deceased. The body was that of Pierre De Rudder, a peasant who had been miraculously cured in the sanctuary of Our Lady in Oostakker. The story of his cure was well known in Belgium and abroad: a falling tree had broken both the tibia and fibula of Pierre's left leg in 1867. Unfortunately, the wound did not heal for eight years and doctors advised an amputation. Pierre, however, refused to do so and suffered through the pain caused by the festering wound (including a gap between the bones of almost three centimetres), from which small frag-

* The author would like to thank Kaat Wils and Henk de Smaele for their comments on previous versions of this text.

1 Van Hoestenberghe, Royer and Deschamps, 'Récit', 559.

ments of dead bone occasionally emerged. A visit to the replica Lourdes grotto in Oostakker in April 1875 eventually brought him the instantaneous cure for which he had hoped and prayed.

The exceptional nature of his recovery made Pierre one of Lourdes' most famous *miraculés* and the object of a fervent debate, which also continued after his death from pneumonia in March 1898.[2] To strengthen Pierre's case, several medical examinations were conducted before and after his death.[3] Two of these were done at the request of Lourdes and tell us something about the importance attached to Pierre's cure. Dr Boissarie, head of the Lourdes Bureau of Medical Verifications, made the first request in 1893, only a few days after Charcot had published his *La foi qui guérit*. The doctor believed that a confirmation of the exceptional character of Pierre's cure could help to refute accusations made by those sceptical of Lourdes. Pierre's cure was an 'organic' case of healing 'far from the intoxicating crowds of Lourdes' and, therefore, according to Suzanne Kaufman, 'invulnerable to the usual accusations made by anticlerical doctors, especially charges of suggestion'.[4] Fourteen years later, in 1907, the Lourdes sanctuary wanted to celebrate the fiftieth anniversary of the apparitions of Bernadette with the canonical recognition of the most famous miracles. Among these they listed De Rudder's cure – thus, a canonical examination began.[5]

Pierre's legs figured prominently in the Lourdes campaigns and the medical discussions. The most famous image of him (printed in devotional and medical treatises) is a case in point: the picture shows him with his trouser legs pulled up, displaying his healthy, bare legs. More 'scientific' images of his legs circulated as well, and X-rays were taken in 1897. As X-rays were only invented in 1895, Pierre's are most probably among the first well-known examples.[6] The visible 'proof' of Pierre's cure was also turned into tangible proof. After that early morning in Jabbeke in May 1899, plaster casts of his bones were made and put on display in Lourdes (in the museum) and in Oostakker

2 Deschamps, *Le cas de Pierre De Rudder*, 73-110; *Le cas de De Rudder*, 13. On the medical discussions and even the wages, see also Kaufman, *Consuming Visions*, 184-193.

3 For example, in 1875, 1893, 1899 and 1907-1908. The first one was conducted immediately after Pierre's cure by Dr Van Hoestenberghe (the Jabbeke doctor to the poor who had regularly treated Pierre) and at the request of the bishop of Bruges, Mgr Faict. Another occurred in 1899, undertaken by Dr Dechamps, S.J. and Dr Jos Van Hoestenberghe, S.J. (son of the doctor from Stahille) from May until August 1899, after Pierre's bones had become available for closer examination. On the examinations, see Van Hoestenberghe, Royer and Deschamps, 'Récit', 555. The three mentioned here were not the only ones, see De Meester, *La guérison miraculeuse*, 10-11.

4 Kaufman, *Consuming Visions*, 182.

5 The examination even included surgical experiments on the corpse of an octogenarian by Dr Rubbrecht and Dr Nelis, attended by Deschamps (demanding first a partial and later the complete fracture of the bones). De Meester, *De wonderbare genezing*, 191-193 and Id., *La guérison miraculeuse*, 5.

6 De Meester, *De wonderbare genezing*, 34.

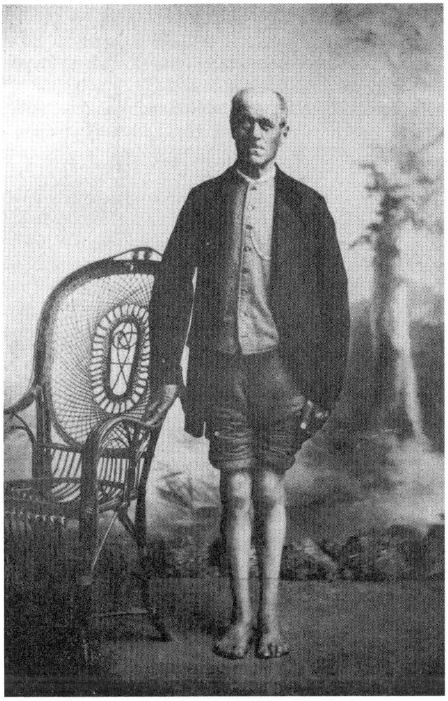

Pierre De Rudder after his cure.
[*L. Van Hoestenberghe, E. Royer and A. Deschamps. 'Récit et étude d'une guérison subite de fracture'.* Revue des questions scientifiques, *October 1899, 517*]

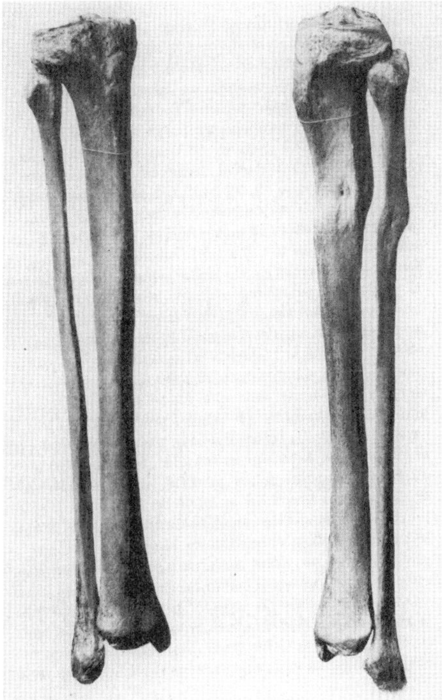

Bones of Pierre De Rudder.
[*L. Van Hoestenberghe, E. Royer and A. Deschamps. 'Récit et étude d'une guérison subite de fracture'.* Revue des questions scientifiques, *October 1899, 527*]

(in 1936, near the grotto). Moreover, the bones were physically examined and meticulously studied by doctors,[7] sparking new debate.[8]

Even 75 years after the cure, the bones (preserved by the diocese of Bruges) still drew attention. In the summer of 1950, Dr L. Elaut examined the original bones, ordered X-rays and concluded that the fibula and tibia of the left leg each showed a callus. In his opinion, the bone fractures had been healed by the creation of new bone material, a 'banal and natural' healing process. However, considering the complexity of the wound, as well as the eight years it had refused to heal and the resulting loss of bone fragments, the speed with which the leg finally healed was anything but natural.[9]

7 When a group of French Catholic doctors gathered for their annual meeting on 21 October 1900, they examined a cast of the bones. The doctors belonged to the Catholic Medical Society of Saint Luc, Saint Côme and Saint Damien. De Meester, *De wonderbare genezing*, 206.

8 Also in France, Germany, the Netherlands and Italy. De Meester, *La guérison miraculeuse*, 13.

9 Elaut, 'Mirakel en wetenschap', 96, 99, 103.

Why start this book with the afterlife of the bones of a *miraculé*? Pierre's case is one among many in which discussions centred on the question of how to 'read' a body. His story illustrates how a body that behaves in a way that is 'out of the ordinary' could stimulate discussion and be used as physical 'proof' by opponents, who interpreted the facts differently, resorting to new tests and producing new evidence (e.g. by using the newest techniques such as X-rays). The demarcation line was not necessarily drawn between science and religion: the subsequent examinations illustrate the Catholic Church's use of medical expertise in order to strengthen a case and respond to new scientific hypotheses. Moreover, among the secular doctors, there was no consensus about how to interpret the findings – there was no unanimity in confronting the religious interpretation of the phenomena. Fervent medical debates frequently developed and stimulated the search for medical proof and explanations. As for the latter, doctors sometimes saw 'faith' as a beneficial influence in the healing process, as Charcot's *La foi qui guérit* exemplifies.

Contrast, collaboration and cross-overs

Within this book, exceptional bodies such as Pierre's will be used as vehicles to look at the developments in two fields of knowledge: science and religion. However, the emphasis is not solely placed on the debates within one or the other epistemological system (science, religion), but also on the cross-overs and collaborations between them. 'Knowledge', promoted and circulated in one 'field of knowledge', might respond to and benefit from developments in other fields of knowledge.[10] This book explores how the evolutions within science and religion influenced each other (e.g. scientific studies of new types of religious phenomena; or references to new medical diagnoses in religious commissions), a productive interaction that has been hidden from view until now. This omission can be linked to some historiographical traditions.

The first issue concerns the historiography of nineteenth- and twentieth-century religion has long been characterized by a certain lack of interest in these mystical phenomena. This is, in part, due to the fact that historians regarded them as a form of 'irrational' religiosity; an anachronism best ignored in the history of 'modern' (and thus 'rational') religion.[11] Interestingly, one of the major reasons why these exceptional bodies re-entered modern religious history was precisely the Church's use of medical expertise in these matters.[12] Secondly, the history of science and, more specifically, the history of psychia-

10 Sarasin, 'Was ist Wissensgeschichte?', 164 and 167.

11 See also the recent comments by Hartney ('Finding a Place', 272) in his historiographical overview of works on divination.

12 See e.g. the work of Jacalyn Duffin, *Medical Miracles*; and Jason Szabo, 'Seeing is Believing?'.

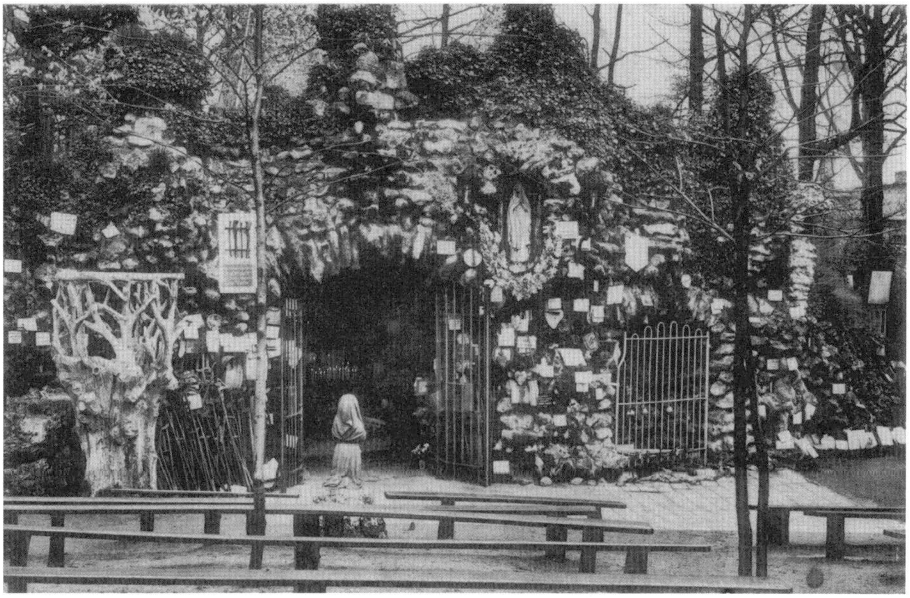

Postcard from Oostakker: the Lourdes grotto and a cast of the bones of Pierre De Rudder. [*Leuven, KADOC-KU Leuven*]

try, have long been dominated by a narrative in which rational science triumphed over obscure religious beliefs and clerical authority. There was little to no room for a less oppositional approach or an interest in the inspiration that medical professionals might have drawn from religion.[13] Religion was approached as a potential source of illness rather than as a genuine intellectual challenge.

The late nineteenth-century 'pathologization' of religion is particularly well researched. With the rise of the nation-states, the emerging medical subdisciplines were linked to the state and differentiated from the 'other' epistemological realm dominant at the time: religion. Scholars such as Jan Goldstein (working on France) and Manuel Borutta (on Germany and Italy) have shown how, in this process, religious phenomena such as stigmata were pathologized, reduced to purely physiological phenomena and hence 'secularized'. Defining stigmata or ecstasy, for example, as 'pathological', meant moulding them into 'expectable', explainable phenomena; into recognizable symptomatologies and predictable prognoses (e.g. various stages of fits). They were, in other words, 'normalized' and standardized. Diagnosing such events implied exercising medical power, claiming 'authority' over the definition of the corporeal phenomena.

Such re-evaluations also had political implications: the nineteenth-century redefinition of 'hysteria' as a neurological disorder was linked to anti-

13 Westerink, 'Demonic Possession', 335.

Catholicism and the creation of liberal government. This meant that defining a religious experience as 'hysterical' also implied questioning the Church and religion. Not only were contemporary events studied from this perspective, but also, taking a universalist approach, saints, witches and the possessed, who were all retrospectively re-evaluated and described in pathological terms, suggesting that exaggerated religiosity could damage one's physical health.[14] However, this focus on 'religious' symptoms, iconography and motives also had the paradoxical result that these medics 're-embedded Catholicism into their scientific practice'.[15] For example, some of the bodily movements of the patients were described in religious terms, such as 'crucifixion' and 'ecstasy'. The bodies of these patients were subject to the gaze in public settings (such as public lectures or books), documented with new technologies (such as photographs) and consequently became part of a culture of 'spectacular visibility'.[16]

However, it is necessary to mention some caveats before proceeding further. Firstly, it is important to emphasize the chronological specificity of this stance and the intensity of the debate. The French Third Republic is the prototypical setting of such discussions and of a professionalizing psychiatric discipline wrenching itself free from the involvement of the Church and clergy. Nevertheless, scholars such as Jacques Maître and Hervé Guillemain, focusing on the case of France, document a more harmonious collaboration between medical and clerical professionals in both the early nineteenth and early twentieth centuries.[17] Philippe Pinel, for example, never considered that his own work opposed reigning ideas on possession. Moreover, his 'moral treatment' drew on pastoral models and referred to the positive and negative effects of religious authority.[18] Pinel also differentiated between religious ideas and practices that had a negative effect (e.g. rigorist Jansenism that

14 Borutta, 'Das Andere der Moderne', 66; Goldstein, 'The Hysteria Diagnosis', 210; Minois, *L'Église et la science*, 299; Velle, 'De geneeskunde en de R.K. Kerk', 11; Edelman, *Les métamorphoses de l'hystérique*, 208. For critical views on the 'medicalization of society', see e.g. Nys et al., *De zieke natie*, 13.

15 Harris, 'The "unconscious" and Catholicism in France', 331 and 338; see also Gilman, 'The Image of the Hysteric', 372.

16 Didi-Huberman, *Invention de l'hystérie*, 13, 18; Langlois, 'La photographie', 328; Christian, 'L'œil de l'esprit', 7; Gilman, 'The Image of the Hysteric', 352-353. They were so well known that they even generated a new style of performance in the French cabarets ('chanteuses épileptiques') and cinema, see Gordon, *De Charcot à Charlot*. On the limits of photographic representation of the hysteric (specific actions of single patients) in regard to drawings and etchings, see Gilman, *Seeing the Insane*, 198.

17 Maître, 'De Bourneville à nos jours'; Guillemain, *Diriger les consciences*, 101.

18 Westerink, 'Demonic Possession', 336; Goldstein, *Console and Classify*, 85-87, 201, 209. Ironically, the nuns and monks involved in mental care reclaimed and accentuated 'the religious elements that had originally helped to inspire the moral treatment, using the medical-scientific authority that validated moral means in order to subvert that same authority'.

could lead to despair; extreme unction) and those with a positive outcome (e.g. the Jesuits' more lenient stance on sin).[19]

Similarly, Ann Goldberg's study of German asylums in the early nineteenth century indicates that the most important fault line was not between science and religion but between excessive religion (as represented in the neo-orthodoxy of the time) and rationalist religion. In her opinion, the anticlericalism that had played such an important role for the French alienists did not apply to Germany. 'German psychiatrists (primarily rationalists) saw religion not as a competing force, but in its proper rationalist form as a bulwark against mental and social disorder' and they continued to employ clerics in the institutional care of mental illness.[20]

Moreover, in spite of this focus on Catholicism by the above-mentioned scholars, ideas on the correlation between extreme forms of religious experience and illness were not limited to one denomination or to the modern era. Jan Goldstein has remarked that the association with hysteria seems to have been so commonplace that in eighteenth-century England, 'Jon Wesley was to volunteer a pre-emptive that his Methodist converts beset by uncontrollable paroxysms were not hysterical'. In other words, the French doctor Jean-Martin Charcot (who redefined hysteria), and his colleagues at the psychiatric hospital of la Salpêtrière, fit into an older tradition.[21] Nevertheless, diagnosing certain religious phenomena as illnesses assisted the emerging disciplines of neurology and psychiatry to substantiate their claims of medical expertise.[22]

The second historiographical issue, as Marques and Guillemain emphasize, concerns the importance of historicizing the religious phenomena and the experiences that were the object of these studies. The beginning of the nineteenth century in France was an era of publicly present, self-declared religious and political messiahs, mystics and prophets – a phenomenon described as 'theomania'.[23] The Church was also critical of this type of religiosity.[24] Similar ly, Hervé Guillemain has demonstrated how the religious conjuncture of the second half of the nineteenth century – Rome's loss of its temporal power, the trauma of the Commune – created an atmosphere in France in which an apocalyptic Catholicism could thrive.[25] Phenomena such as the 'mal de Morzine', demonic possession and stigmatics drew attention and, as Herman Westerink

19 Goldstein, *Console and Classify*, 213.
20 Goldberg, *Sex, Religion*, 48.
21 Goldstein, 'The Hysteria Diagnosis', 238-239.
22 Hayward, 'Demonology', 38; Westerink, 'Demonic Possession', 337; Goldberg, *Sex, Religion*, 50.
23 Marques, 'Mystique, politique et maladie mentale', 47. See also Bowman, 'Une lecture politique de la folie religieuse', 84.
24 For similar trends in the German states and how they were linked up with new bourgeois ideas about self-control, see Goldberg, *Sex, Religion*, 42.
25 Guillemain, *Diriger les consciences*, 137; Marques, 'Mystique, politique et maladie mentale', 49.

has pointed out, 'it was in this context that psychiatrists became increasingly interested in a range of strange corporeal symptom formations, notably the phenomenon of convulsions which they began to describe as prototypical of hysteria'.[26] Nevertheless, the cases singled out by the medical professionals were given more importance than the clergy attached to them and, as discussed more elaborately below, in order to counter these currents, the Church also adopted pathologizing strategies – thus making their own contribution to the secularization of madness.[27]

While most scholars working on the intersection of the history of the body and religious history have focused on the Middle Ages, an interest in the modern era – a period of the revitalization of and innovation in corporeal religious practices[28] – is steadily increasing. Important impulses have come from scholars working in women's and gender studies, who have paid special attention to the role of the body in the construction of gender and in claims to authority, linking these to religious ideas and practices (e.g. 'vicarious suffering', 'holy' anorexia).[29] Considering the modern cases, it is important to point out that there were various stances taken on the importance of various corporeal phenomena (such as inedia, stigmata, ecstasy, levitation, visions). As the popular support of stigmatics and fasting women indicates, some believed the physical phenomena of mysticism to be proof of divine grace and a sign of holiness.[30] Nonetheless, the Catholic Church's official stance on these corporeal phenomena was far more critical, as proven by the eighteenth-century work, *De servorum Dei beatificazione et beatorum canonizatione* by Prospero Lambertini, later Pope Benedict XIV. He emphasized that such corporeal phenomena were not sufficient reason to perceive someone as holy, attaching greater importance to their virtues.[31]

26 Westerink, 'Demonic Possession', 337.

27 Guillemain, *Diriger les consciences*, 137; Marques, 'Mystique, politique et maladie mentale', 49.

28 Pulz, 'Vorbemerkung', 8, 10.

29 Kane, '"She offered herself up"'; Bynum, 'Holy Anorexia', 243; Scheer, 'Das Medium hat ein Geschlecht', 170, 177; Schneider, 'Marienerscheinungen', 106. In cases like that of Louise Beck, the corporeal experience figured as a basis for claims of religious authority – their bodies functioning as religious media. See Weiß, *Weisungen aus dem Jenseits?* Scholars working on modern religion emphasize the importance of studying the historicized body as an 'experiencing agent'. Such analyses stress how experiences contributed to the construction of reality and hence also to the interpretations of the divine. Scheer, 'Verspielte Frömmigkeit', 387.

30 According to scholars such as Nicole Priesching, Otto Weiß and Monique Scheer, the predominance of women among these 'mystics' can be explained by referring to the gender ideology of the era that linked women to corporeality. Women expressing Christian ideals (even representing Christ's body) via their own bodies thus accords with the conceptions of their contemporaries. Priesching, 'Mystikerinnen'; Weiß, 'Stigmata', 119; Scheer, 'Das Medium hat ein Geschlecht', 169, 177.

31 Pulz, 'Vorbemerkung', 7; Weiß, 'Stigmata', 112, 120 and Zumholz, 'Die Resistenz des katholischen Milieus', 223.

The case of the Catholic doctor Imbert-Gourbeyre illustrates how in the late nineteenth century the Vatican wanted to encourage a more sceptical stance towards these exceptional bodies. The doctor was criticized for his study of stigmatics, which included an elaborate appraisal of the exterior signs (rather than the virtues of the person) and a description of them as saints.[32] The Church expected the doctors to act as medical experts rather than aspiring theologians and frequently called upon their expertise. Studies on canonization processes, on the reception of stigmatics, or the recognition of miraculous cures,[33] have demonstrated how the Catholic Church instigated and referred to medical examinations. The importance of medical findings, the reliance on medical expertise in gauging the 'authenticity' of the phenomena in question, has been called the 'medicalization of the miracle' and has primarily been linked to the nineteenth century.[34] However, as Jacalyn Duffin has pointed out in her work on canonization processes, from 1588 onwards, the Catholic Church paid increasing attention to physical healing supported by medical testimony.[35] The discussions in which the Church became embroiled did provide extra reason for caution and stimulated interest in medical examinations of cases believed to be 'exceptional'. It was thought that no well-examined and well-documented case could be easily rejected by enemies of the Church.[36] The various cases illustrate how the Church kept track of new diagnoses and evolutions in the medical field. Those who collaborated with the Bureau of Medical Verifications in Lourdes,[37] for example, willingly admitted that many of the patients who came to Lourdes were 'hysterics', and they even developed their own definition of 'hysteria'.[38] Moreover, as noted in the story of Pierre De Rudder, the Bureau increasingly focused on the miraculous cures of organic lesions when theories of suggestion became more popular.[39]

As the display of Pierre's bones in Lourdes and Oostakker indicates, visible 'proof' was of central importance. *Miraculé(e)s* were lined up in public processions, but also put on display at gatherings organized by the Bureau – as living proof of their cure and 'normality'.[40] Similarly, ideas on religious

32 Guillemain, *Diriger les consciences*, 141.

33 Duffin, *Medical Miracles*; e.g. in discussions of the Belgian stigmatic Louise Lateau, Lachapelle, 'Between Miracle and Sickness', 88.

34 Foucault, *The Birth of the Clinic*; Szabo, 'Seeing is Believing?', 211; Desmazières, 'Psychology against Medicine?', 1192 ('the medical intrusion into a field traditionally controlled by theology'). See also Amiotte-Suchet, 'Tous égaux devant Dieu?', 246.

35 Duffin, *Medical Miracles*, 35.

36 Edelman, *Les métamorphoses de l'hystérique*, 215; Maître, 'De Bourneville à nos jours', 772.

37 Szabo, 'Seeing is Believing?'; Harris, 'Les miraculés de Lourdes'.

38 Edelman, *Les métamorphoses de l'hystérique*, 216-217. See also the work of Catholic doctors on the psychology of stigmatics, Weiß, 'Stigmata', 120; Id., 'Seherinnen und Stigmatisierte', 53.

39 Guillemain, *Diriger les consciences*, 231.

40 Kaufman, *Consuming Visions*, 115-117.

'madness' also had an impact on the images of the modern 'mystics'. Claude Langlois has argued that the images used in the promotion of Bernadette or Therese of Lisieux were carefully selected and staged to emphasize their 'normality'.[41] Charcot had to dig deeper into the past to find visual examples for his *Les démoniaques dans l'art*. In this book, he traced cases of demonic possession in works of art from the fifth to the eighteenth century, and he postulated, on the grounds of the postures the demoniacs assumed, that they had in fact been hysterics.[42]

The new means of medical visualization also had an impact. A particularly telling example is that referred to by William Christian in his study of the Spanish visionaries of Ezquioga. After explaining how the carefully selected images of the visionaries in trances resembled older devotional images, Christian notes how the Jesuit José Antonio Laburu aimed to minimize the impact that these photographic representation of the visionaries had on their supporters. To discredit the visionaries, he filmed two of the leading figures and showed the film in fast-motion, 'pour qu'ils ressemblent à ceux qu'il avait pris d'internés dans un asile psychiatrique'.[43]

Moreover, religious ideas changed in response to new medical findings. Anthony Ossa-Richardson's work on chaplains in English lunatic asylums documents how discussions about how to read passages of the New Testament were linked to psychiatric ideas, and not only by elite scholars. Questions arose about whether or not the Evangelists had made a distinction between lunatics and 'demoniacs', and if the demoniacs that Jesus cured were in fact madmen and epileptics.[44] Similarly, in his study of Fundamentalist and Pentacostalist discussions about demonology, Rhodri Hayward has pointed out that their ideas about possession and conversion changed and their 'writings drew upon medical and psychiatric sources ranging widely from Pastorian germ theory to Jacksonian neurology'. In short, they 'incorporated contemporary psychiatric, neurological, and epidemiologic knowledge as part of a general attempt to make sense of their supernatural experience'.[45]

At the same time, medical scholars were fascinated by the effect that religion (and more generally 'faith') could have on the psyches and bodies of their patients. As noted, early nineteenth-century German psychiatrists thereby differentiated between the healthy influence of religious guidance and the

41 '... normalité de la voyante et banalité pieuse de ses gestes publiques, ici; et là, chez Thérèse, dissociation totale entre le corps, insignifiant, sinon comme support d'une identité biographique, et donc livré sans peine à la photographie, et l'âme, qui seule a une histoire'. Langlois, 'La photographie', 332.

42 Charcot and Richer, *Les démoniaques dans l'art*; Goldstein, *Console and Classify*, 370-371.

43 Christian, 'L'œil de l'esprit', 12.

44 Ossa-Richardson, 'Possession or Insanity?', 568.

45 Hayward, 'Demonology', 37 and 39, 54, e.g. in relation to demonic activity: 'They described a process whereby demons lodged themselves in nervous ganglia of the neck and spinal column in order to corrupt the subject's personality'.

negative effects of religious fanaticism. A similar differentiation can be traced in the work of their French colleagues. While Pinel's 'moral treatment' was a secularized variation on the theme of religious guidance and built on its comforting and consoling character, Pinel also believed in the negative effects of religion, which he saw at work in cases where the patient's passions did not agree with religious scruples.[46] The positive effect also features prominently in Charcot's *La foi qui guérit* – an ambiguous title that, as Jacqueline Lalouette has pointed out, leaves undecided the question of whether 'foi' should be understood in a theological sense or more generally as faith and confidence. In fact, in the text: 'Charcot confirme que *faith healing* religieuse et laïque ne peuvent être dédoublées, que l'une et l'autre aboutissent à la même opération cérébrale produisant des effets identiques'.[47]

The book's ambitions and limits

The chapters comprising this book discuss the production and circulation of knowledge stimulated by bodies behaving in a manner that is out of the ordinary, and focuses on expertise and/or scientific authority over a period ranging from the early nineteenth century until the mid-twentieth century. As this brief overview has already indicated, religion and science developed through a process of interaction: a changing religious climate (and the concomitant new religious currents) provided new cases for study; religious phenomena inspired new medical approaches (e.g. about the healing power of faith); new medical findings could be adopted to oppose new messiahs; and medical imagery came to inspire the campaigns of opponents of aberrant religious currents. The following chapters contribute to the study of this interaction by broadening the perspective in several ways.

Firstly, most of the work that has been done on the interaction between science and religion has focused on France. To what extent was that country exemplary? Jan Goldstein, for example, has noted that the tensions between religion and psychiatry were not as strong in Great Britain as they were in France.[48] How important were the national contexts and local factors in the discussions between medical and religious authorities? The following chapters not only look into France but also address the English, Portuguese, Austrian and Belgian contexts.

46 Similarly, Esquirol believed that religious passions could lead to monomania, Marques, 'Mystique, politique et maladie mentale', 40, 51-52; Jackson, *Care of the Psyche*, 187. For the German psychiatrists, see the work of Goldberg, *Sex, Religion*.

47 Lalouette, referred to in Bonduelle, Gelfand and Goetz, *Charcot*, 224. See e.g. the impact of Lourdes on ideas about the influence of religion on organic structure, Guillemain, *Diriger les consciences*, 230.

48 Goldstein, 'Psychiatry'.

Moreover, some of the authors contributing to this volume have adopted a transnational perspective and look at the circulation of knowledge (and its implications) between France and its protectorates; or the Continent and the United States. Did the discovery of exceptional corporeal phenomena in the colonies stimulate new debates in the motherland, and did the imported and local systems of knowledge clash? What was the impact of transnational (scientific and religious) networks?

The following chapters also address levels of circulation of this knowledge in contexts other than those where experts (theologians and scientists) were active. In order to define the impact of new knowledge, it is important to look at the 'consumers' and the effect that this knowledge had on their ideas of religion or science. Studies on the reception of nineteenth-century mystics have demonstrated that Catholic contemporaries could have quite different ideas about the corporeal phenomena and did not always follow Rome's guidelines. Addressing various levels of circulation of knowledge and adopting a broader geographical perspective also allows us to ask questions about the use of knowledge in identity/community constructions and strategies of 'othering'. Research on the Catholic alienist, August Morel, for example, has shown that he believed that epidemics of religious delirium were more frequent in Protestant countries and in India among the Buddhists, and that he linked them to his ideas about degeneration.[49] However, did this differentiation only play a role at the scholarly level?

The conceptualizations of corporeal phenomena, epistemology and the importance of scientific specialization and fragmentation are central issues in the first two chapters of this volume, both of which focus on the medical field. In the first chapter, Maria Heidegger studies the treatment of religious pathologies in an early nineteenth-century Tyrolean institute, where about half of the patient files mention an illness that could be linked to religious convictions. Heidegger postulates that rather than starting from a distinction between secular and religious epistemologies, in each case the proponents of the two fields of knowledge negotiated the thin line between a healthy and an unhealthy involvement in religion. The later could be expressed in, for example, convulsions and other bodily movements, which were deemed symptomatic of the illness by the doctors, but for the patients were a sign of diabolic possession. Both religion and medicine – personified in the chaplains and the doctors respectively – were faced with the challenges of religious pathologies. What is more, religious practices (such as confession) and guidance were built into the therapeutic process. While psychiatric and pastoral actors could operate in competition, they also often collaborated in their shared interest in the well-being of the tormented soul.

49 Marques, 'Mystique, politique et maladie mentale', 60.

In her study of France and Austria, Nicole Edelman points to the similarities and differences in the perceptions of exceptional corporeal phenomena by three doctors in the late nineteenth century and early twentieth century. All three, Jean-Marie Charcot, Gustave Boissarie and Sigmund Freud, were trained in 'reading' bodies, they were all familiar with the world of hospitals and were well known beyond their national borders. Nevertheless, they all had quite different ideas about the role of religion in the development of these phenomena (seeing it as a phase or a cause of, or as a remedy for, an affliction).

The following two chapters focus on female lay mystics of the 1870s. The two cases discussed here, the French farmer's wife, Marie Bergadieu, and the English school teacher, Teresa Higginson, both feature prominently in discussions about Catholic identity, but while Marie turned into a symbolic figure for French royalists, Teresa became symbolic of what English Catholics claimed *not* to be. In her chapter on the ecstatic from Fontet, Sofie Lachapelle describes how Marie Bergadieu's body was invested with political and religious meaning, which created commercial possibilities. In those early years of the French Third Republic, Fontet quickly developed into a pilgrimage centre and Marie and her royalist prophecies seemed to confirm the hope of those who still believed in the return of a monarchical system. Marie's popularity benefited from the willingness of physicians to declare her trances genuine and the Church's initially rather cautious stance. Her popularity thrived in a political and religious context in which Marie could function as a symbol of hope. As the Republican system continued to function (also for royalists), the need for this hope soon diminished and Marie's fame vanished.

In her article on the reception of Teresa Higginson, Mary Heimann looks into what the stigmatic meant to both her contemporaries and to the English Catholics of the interwar period, when the cause for Teresa's beatification was launched, triggering fierce debate. Heimann shows how Teresa Higginson's 'extravagantly medieval behaviour' and her 'doctrinally precise' language turned her, in the eyes of her contemporary supporters, into a 'touchstone of eternal Catholic truth in the midst of nineteenth-century modernity and scepticism'. The comparative rarity of her stigmata in Victorian Britain and the other mystical phenomena she claimed to experience helped her popularity. However, when the cause for beatification was launched, Teresa was used as a vehicle through which various ideas about how the Catholic minority ought to present itself were vented. Supporters of the cause emphasized the mystical tradition of Catholic hagiography and the need to 'embrace all that made Catholicism distinctive', while those who opposed her beatification feared that it would bring ridicule to English Catholicism and used medical language to discredit Theresa.

Questions of difference and integration also dominate the next chapter. In her contribution on Catholic America, Paula Kane examines whether the scarcity of mystical phenomena with affective physical effects can be linked to American Catholics' struggle to fit in; to avoid the stigma of a superstitious and anti-scientific Catholicism and overcome the perception of the 'foreignness of Catholicism'. Nevertheless, while some American Catholics minimized the importance of such phenomena, others emphasized the similarities between the American and European cases, and used the few examples to make connections with the Old World Catholics (where such phenomena were on the rise during the nineteenth and twentieth centuries) and contribute to the creation of an international Catholic identity. Kane highlights the transnational aspect of these discussions and points to the significant mediating role of the European clergy, the 'importation' of European debates on 'hysterical' stigmatics and the use of European templates to promote American cases.

The issues of citizenship and nationality also echo through the chapter by Ellen J. Amster, who discusses epistemological struggles in French-colonial Morocco. In this context, she focuses on the *majnun*, an example of the male Islamic saints 'whose knowledge of God' manifested 'as exceptional corporeal phenomena'. Capable of influencing the bodies of others (as a site of veridiction and healing), the *majnun* also illustrated his lack of ego through his own body and repulsive antinomian behaviour. While he had only been a marginal figure in Islamic hagiography, after the French conquest the *majnun* became 'a fundamentally irrational Islamic figure whose unassimilable character opposed western civilization'. The modernist and positivist French physicians and sociologists pathologized these mystical phenomena as hysteria or neurosis. Similarly, the Moroccan nationalist movement (1930-1956) called for modern French medicine and attacked saint healing as heretical, savage and unscientific.

The final two contributions primarily focus on the use of scientific and religious knowledge in asserting the authenticity and credibility of religious experiences and their corporeal expression. Tiago Pires Marques examines cases of Marian apparitions (Fatima, 1917) and victim souls (Alexandrina of Balasar) in Portugal in the first half of the twentieth century. While emphasizing the importance of the changing content and context of psychiatry (processes of institutionalization and de-politicization in the 1920s-1940s), he points out how medical knowledge was woven into religious experience which, 'in turn actualized or helped displace certain scientific themes'. Medical and religious epistemologies did not necessarily stand in opposition to each other. Religious authorities adopted psychiatric terms when arguing for the pathological character of a religious experience (the 'hysterical woman' was a well-known counter-type) and used scientific methods to 'test' whether the visionaries involved were believable subjects, and whether their extraordinary bodies supported the suggestion of divine intervention. The two cases illustrate how 'the modernizing world of miraculous Catholicism integrated scientific dimensions whether as a reality level for consideration (...) or as a competing interpretative frame to combat, negotiate with and virtually co-opt'.

Finally, in her chapter on a series of Marian apparitions in 1930s Belgium, Tine Van Osselaer studies the lay response to the medical examinations of the phenomena. Laypeople alternated between demanding and criticizing the medical examinations. Commenting upon the doctors' experiments at the sites and their examination of the *miraculés*, laypeople referred to medical authority when pleading their case. At the same time, however, they did not hesitate to question the authority and competence of the doctors and call upon the Church's authority when they believed this to be more favourable to their cause.

As this brief introduction indicates, often there was no strict polarization between religion and science, sign or symptom. Pierre's legs, amputated in the pastor's garden and meticulously examined by medical professionals, could easily pass from one field of knowledge to another, generating productive debates. Hopefully, the following pages will do the same.

Acknowledgements

This book is the result of a workshop organized by Tine Van Osselaer, Henk de Smaele and Kaat Wils on 12-14 September 2013 at KADOC, Documentation and Research Centre for Religion, Culture and Society of the KU Leuven. The editors would like to thank the Research Foundation Flanders, KADOC, the research unit Modernity & Society (KU Leuven) and the research unit Cultural History since 1750 (KU Leuven) for their generous support of that meeting.

We owe a great debt to all the scholars who participated in that workshop and those who helped to organize it (especially Wannes Dupont). We were very lucky in finding such a wonderful set of authors who were willing to engage with the comments and suggestions of the editors and, in a later phase, the external referees. We hope the harmonious collaboration reflects in the following pages and are grateful to the KADOC team in helping us to prepare the volume.

THE DEVIL IN THE MADHOUSE

ON THE TREATMENT OF RELIGIOUS PATHOLOGIES IN EARLY PSYCHIATRY, TYROL, 1830-1850

MARIA HEIDEGGER

> The delusion of demonic possession persists all the more obstinately when it has previously been reinforced by clerics; often – especially when [the patient's] condition is being discussed – it involves epileptic seizures, which give the impression of something alive coursing through the body; at the same time, she complains of tension and pain in the head.[1]

These were the words set down by an assistant physician in a so-called 'lunatic record' ['Irrenprotokoll'] in August 1843 to describe the condition of patient Josepha S*, admitted to the Imperial Provincial Insane Asylum in Hall, in the county of Tyrol, with a diagnosis of 'lunacy in a hysterical individual'. Regarding her 'treatment', he noted: 'She is kept busy with sewing, knitting, and spinning to occupy her attention, required to obey house rules, and in particular commended to the psychological influence of the Rev[erend] Chaplain.'[2] Record entries such as this one crystallize the key aspects of the issues explored in this article. With admission and the creation of a patient file, the character of the mental suffering had already been decided; the observed symptoms were taken as evidence of illness. Josepha S*'s symptoms would soon be viewed as pathological in the context of a diagnosis of delusion, and the history of her suffering would accordingly be interpreted,

1 Historisches Archiv des Landeskrankenhauses Hall in Tirol [HA LKH], Krankenakten Frauen 1845, Josepha S* [Aufnahmebuch] I/[Kopfzahlnummer] 204, Irrenprotokolle.

2 Ibid.

catalogued, and managed. Her diagnosis – 'lunacy and hysteria' – appeared conspicuously at the top of her file; in Tyrol, the diagnosis of 'demon mania', so popular elsewhere, was rare in the early decades of the nineteenth century.[3] In these parts, it seems, the devil was banned even from diagnoses. From both a medical and administration perspective, the institution responsible for the Catholic crown land of Tyrol considered 'the Evil Enemy' to exist in the disordered imagination of the patient, in her delusion, which was inevitably linked to her individual experience.[4] And this delusion – the patient's experience of being possessed – represented a therapeutic challenge to be taken seriously and which (from the vantage of the physician) clearly warranted admission to a modern mental hospital. At the same time, the psycho-medical and curative landscape of this period was variegated, including alternative interventions by spiritual healers, trips to health spas, and pilgrimages. Thus, in the record entry cited here, the physician lamented the patient's worsening condition under the previous harmful influence of a cleric. Moreover, this case alludes to a rivalry within the administratively reshaped landscape of care owing to the establishment of the mental hospital. Yet the record also mentions collaboration with the hospital's spiritual healers as part of the patient's therapy.

The physician who reported on the condition of Josepha S* accepted objectively visible signs as interpreted phenomena, namely, convulsions, and categorized them in the context of an appropriate medical neo-interpretation of such phenomena in the context of hysterical symptoms. Yet he also briefly referred to the self-awareness of the sufferer herself, and a subjective account of the symptoms was inscribed in the file. In addition, the file contains the obligatory enumeration of diverse somatic complaints, interpreted as medical symptoms.[5] Last but not least, the treatment was sketched in terms of contemporary psychic and moral curative methods, which often included collaboration with the asylum's chaplain acting as a kind of spiritual healer.

The early psychiatric medical records of the Tyrolean mental hospital from 1830 suggest an intensified religiosity during the period under study. Nonetheless, the occurrence of religious pathologies in this context is hard to pinpoint statistically owing to conceptual selectivity and inconsistent terminology, and to the dynamic course of disease. In the early days of institutionalized psychiatry the area of concern was assigned various labels, and consequently also differently contextualized and treated. However, a random evaluation of 200 patient files from 1830 to 1850 subjected to detailed textual

3 On the psychiatric adaptation and 'demystification' of possession in the form of a medical diagnosis of 'demon mania' with relevant citations by Busch (1833), Esquirol (1838), Ideler (1837), and Flemming (1844), see Kocherscheidt, *Deutsche Irrenärzte und Irrenseelsorger*, 31-34.

4 Glatzel, *Melancholie und Wahnsinn*, 76.

5 On the medical difference between signs and symptoms, see Nordqvist, 'What are symptoms? What are signs?'.

analysis indicates that 40 out of 100 men and more than 50 out of 100 women suffered one way or another from desperate sadness over their own salvation, fears of damnation, religious melancholy, visions, or possession. The importance of this finding from a history of mentalities perspective forms the basis for my investigation into the treatment of religious pathologies and the historical relationship between pastoral care and early institutional psychiatry, in connection with a more comprehensive research project on 'Caring for the Soul' in the first half of the nineteenth century.

Using exemplary patient files as a starting point, I will focus here on day-to-day asylum practice during the period under study. Through this focus on therapy, I will elucidate how theological and medical discourse around religious pathologies was incorporated into the specific examination of individual suffering. Of particular interest are the repercussions of the emerging confrontation between the overlapping fields of theology and medicine in the mid-nineteenth century – evident in the asylum physician's critique of Josepha S*'s treatment by a clergyman – on everyday therapeutic practice. In cases of religious melancholy or delusion, physicians invoked historically and contextually embedded semiotic knowledge that interpreted signs as significant medical indications designating mental illness, and consequently described subjective symptoms with reference to a medical body. Apropos of everyday practice, the question of treatment-relevant knowledge also arises. In this article I wish to assert that what separates religion and psychiatry in the modern mental hospital is not so much a division between secular and spiritual fields of knowledge. Rather, it is the case-by-case renegotiation of borders between healthy and disordered forms of religiosity carried out by different actors within these two fields of knowledge, which forced both religion and medicine to confront the contemporary challenge of religious pathologies.

Knowledge claims: the challenge of modernity

The establishment of a medical-cure-based mental hospital in Hall, a small town east of the Tyrolean city of Innsbruck, in September 1830 coincided with the end of an initial wave of 'modern' healing institutions in German-speaking countries.[6] Dirk Blasius maintained some time ago that the establishment of such healing institutions – as opposed, for example, to specialized institutions of care and confinement for the 'insane' – was motivated by a new and optimistic belief in the possibility of curing diseased minds.[7] That conviction notwithstanding, the primary condition for recovery (according to the con-

6 Heidegger and Seifert, 'Nun ist aber der Zweck einer Irrenanstalt Heilung'.
7 See Blasius, *'Einfache Seelenstörung'*, 19.

temporary belief of physicians and health officials) was appropriate accommodation in a healing institution and, crucially, a corresponding administrative categorization of inmates as medically 'curable' or 'incurable' along with a distinction between 'dangerous' and 'harmless'. These distinctions were considered individually for each case, and the competence regarding evaluation – a key aspect of the whole process of medicalization with respect to insanity – was exclusively the province of physicians and surgeons commissioned by the admitting authorities. The asylum physicians at Hall considered themselves to be the more competent and experienced physicians, and the new specialists for all forms of mental illness. As such, they took note of these medical case histories, opinions, and 'parere medici' and interweaved them with their own individual 'lunatic histories', which became part of the patient file. The Hall asylum thus acquired legitimacy on the basis of a medical interpretation of signs and symptoms made both before and on admission to the hospital, and again at the summary conclusion of each case history. As ideally conceived, the interpretation should focus on the treatment of curable (or suicidal and dangerous) patients. Such an orientation went hand in hand with increased efforts at analytical categorization of mental diseases, and was ever more closely linked with the claims of the fledgling field of psychiatry to science, in the sense of a clinical doctrine based on experience and observation. In its relation to the public, too, the asylum presented itself as a privileged place of healing thanks to a new set of experts, the 'mad doctors'.[8]

In looking back at early modern hospital psychiatry, a related process of professionalization and negotiation of knowledge claims is nearly always explained with reference to boundary disputes involving the interpretive power of the church(es) and the traditional skills of the clergy in caring for the mind and in spiritual healing.[9] A contemporary overemphasis on such disputes may even be understandable considering the controversial and competing amateur forms of participation by Catholic clergy in the 'motley' medical market of the early nineteenth century, which authorities succeeded in regulating only with great difficulty.[10] Treatment of the melancholic and depressed by exorcism and benediction continued well into the 1800s as the special domain of the clergy,[11] a circumstance that was regularly criticized and rejected by the mad

8 On the creation of the 'modern' asylum, see Nolte and Fangerau, 'Einleitung'. On the sociohistorical context of mental health reform in the early nineteenth century, see Blasius, *Umgang mit Unheilbarem*.

9 On physicians' complaints about clerical intervention, see Chmielewski, 'Norm und Autonomie'. For a standard reference on spiritual healing in the early modern era, see Lederer, *Madness, Religion and the State*.

10 On medicine between 1750 and 1850 as a 'motley fair', see Brockmeyer, *Selbstverständnisse*, 51-71. For examples of the activities of Tyrolean clerics as homeopaths, see my article: Heidegger, 'Die Seelsorger und ihre homöopathische Hausapotheke'.

11 Stolberg, '"Volksfromme" Heilpraktiken und medikale Alltagskultur', 167.

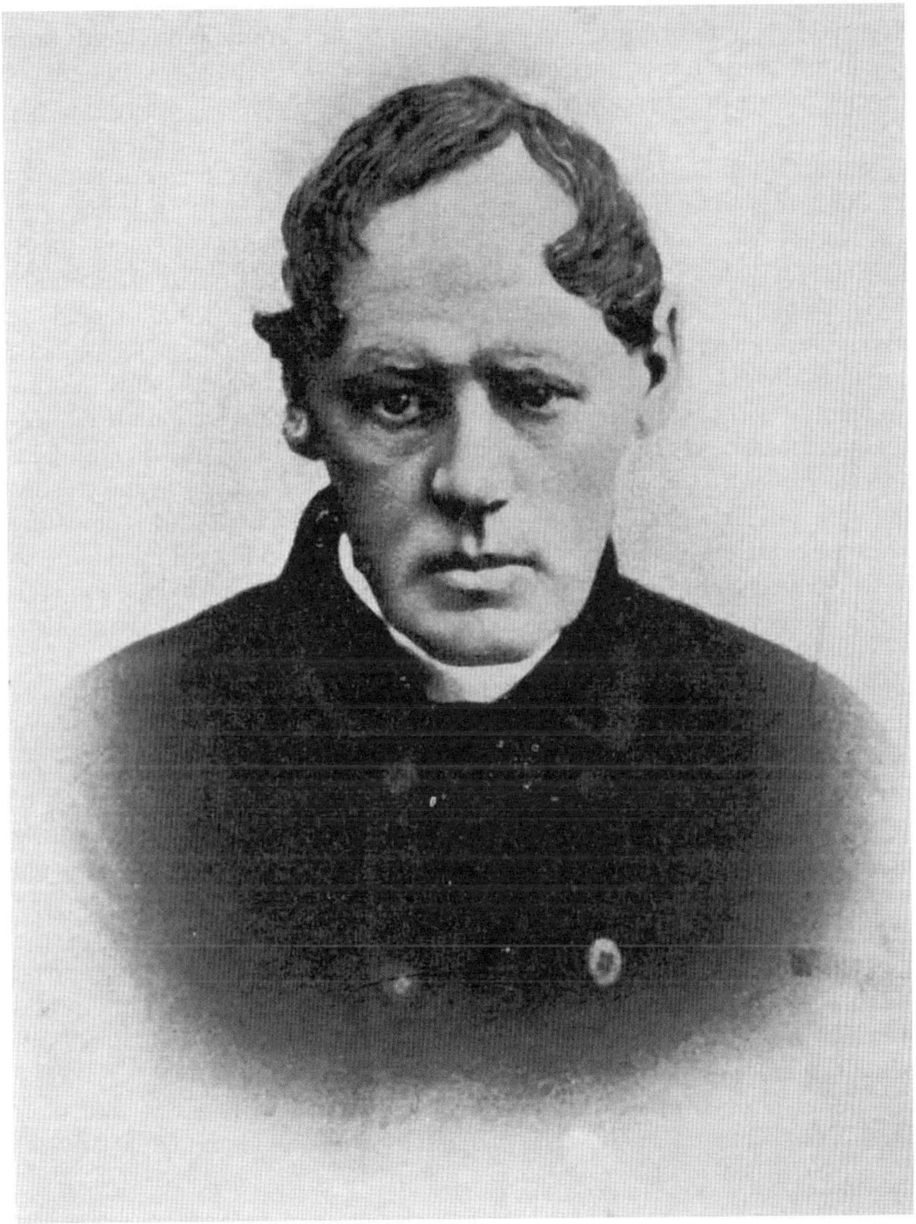

The chaplain of the asylum, Sebastian Ruf (*1802-1877*).
[*Ferdinand Lentner*. Sebastian Ruf. Irrenhaus-Kaplan zu Hall i. T. als Seelenforscher. Ein Beitrag zur Lehre von der Zurechnung im Strafrecht. *Innsbruck, 1902*]

doctors. For contemporaries, these disputes featured quite prominently, and began to wane in importance only in the second half of the 1800s. In terms of the beginnings of psychiatry, however, the specific historical context (i.e., the period leading up to the Austrian revolutions that took place between March 1848 and November 1849, or 'pre-March' period), in which religious pathologies were treated far more diversely, has received relatively little attention.[12] In her landmark book *Sex, Religion, and the Making of Modern Madness* (1999), Ann Goldberg describes how medicine at the start of the nineteenth century revived a much older discourse about the 'mania religiosa' and promoted the asylum as an institutional response to a problem increasingly perceived as a social challenge.[13] Thus, the discourse around religious mania now became an integral part of contemporary professional interests, which in turn meant that the meaning of the phenomenon went far beyond the goal of gaining institutional control over traditionally skilled religious healers in the clashes between religious and secular interpretive frameworks.[14] Now, competing knowledge claims localized not only in the areas of conflict but even more so in the context of day-to-day therapeutic practice, an area in which a common intersection between psychiatric and spiritual healing existed. For although, as Doris Kaufmann writes, the 'mind' or its organ, the brain, was now more widely acknowledged as the 'seat' of insanity, essentially 'a reformulation of the previous theologically possessed soul',[15] the treatment of Josepha S* and her fellow patients did not necessarily involve a corresponding secularization. The newly defined medical sensibility, and thus the interpretation of signs and symptoms as a manifestation of disease, had indeed outgrown the bounds of religion.[16] Nonetheless, the 'modern' asylum at Hall,[17] constructed within the walls of an abandoned Clarissan convent, continued to be based on pre-modern ideas of care and treatment that were deeply embedded in a religious context.[18] To a large extent, the experience of mental suffering and its treatment were determined by religiously shaped perceptions and interpretations not only outside the modern asylum – where most of the mentally ill still sought comfort and help from the clergy – but also within it.

As mentioned above, physicians' professional awareness of, and their professional interest in, religious melancholy and religious mania are un-

12 Angus Gowland notes a comparable lack of research on melancholy in the early modern period: Gowland, 'The Problem of Early Modern Melancholy', 78-79.

13 Goldberg, *Sex, Religion, and the Making of Modern Madness.*

14 Ibid., 51.

15 Kaufmann, *Aufklärung, bürgerliche Selbsterfahrung und die 'Erfindung' der Psychiatrie*, 195. On the philosophical roots of early psychiatry, see Benzenhöfer, *Psychiatrie und Anthropologie*.

16 See Vanja, 'Die Irrenanstalt muss in einer anmutigen Gegend liegen', 23-24.

17 On the term 'modernity' in institutional psychiatry, see Nolte and Fangerau, 'Einleitung'.

18 For an overview, see Vanja, 'Madhouses, Children's Wards, and Clinics'.

derstandable in the context of intensified religiosity during the period under study.[19] Around the middle of the nineteenth century, physicians cited religious despair as the most frequent expression of mental illness in Tyrol. For example, Josef Stolz (1811-1877), medical superintendent and the third director of the mental hospital in Hall, claimed that the Tyrolean farmer would actually be immune to mental illness, but for his Achilles' heel: his deeply religious mind, and too much worrying about salvation.[20] Ten years later, Stolz lamented that a considerable number of melancholics sought religious comfort exclusively, and that many patients thus fell into the hands of visionary clerics. In 'this' country, Stolz argued, melancholic forms of affliction mostly had a religious character, and physicians regularly noted a marked aggravation around religious festivities.[21] Religiosity and religious practices such as confession, church attendance, pilgrimages, and reading religious books were consequently an integral feature of medical observations and case histories. The treatment of religiously tinged pathologies was problematic both from the perspective of contemporary psychiatrists and because this particular group of patients were considered hard to cure.

The prospect of recovery in the context of psychiatric treatment aimed at cure was consequently uncertain. And it was precisely this uncertainty, one might speculate, that motivated a correspondingly strong interest in the early treatment of the insane. In terms of professional legitimacy, the 'business of healing' people with religious melancholy or religious mania was a very risky, and indeed nearly insurmountable, undertaking. In this context, any claims of treatment skills were theoretically closely linked to the challenge of modernity: how to reconcile secular rationality with pathological forms of religiosity. In practice, however, physicians set great store by religious philosophy and a moral lifestyle justified by religion, and alongside other, dietary measures, religion played a decisive role in everyday psychiatry.[22] Johann Tschallener (1783-1855), Hall's second asylum director and medical superintendent, noted, for example, that an essential criterion for a real hope of a successful recovery, apart from a short illness duration, was intact moral health, for only on that basis could an appropriate psycho-pedagogical treatment be introduced.[23] The problem was thus the precarious and difficult-to-define relationship between 'healthy' piety in the sense of a basic requirement for a curative

19 Priesching, *Unter der Geisel Gottes*, 10. On the revival of piety in the nineteenth century, see De Giorgio, 'Die Gläubige'.
20 Stolz, 'Zur fortschreitenden Parese'.
21 Id., 'Aerztlicher Bericht der k. k. Irren-Anstalt zu Hall in Tyrol'.
22 For a concise overview, see Kutzer, 'Die therapeutischen Intentionen in der Irrenanstalt'.
23 Tschallener, *Beschreibung der k. k. Provinzial-Irren-Heilanstalt zu Hall in Tirol*, 301-302.

'dietary' remedy for 'pathological mental disturbances'[24] and the risk of 'eccentric' hyper-religious zeal. The information required for an appropriate assessment should be provided prior to admission to the asylum by means of a 'lunacy examination' conducted by a physician, requiring relevant input from relatives and the parish priest. The latter in particular would be the most reliable and best qualified to provide information regarding whether the patient was a 'religious sceptic' or a 'religious fanatic', a 'free spirit whose orthodox, naively fervent faith was a source of disturbing views', or 'perhaps one who had [encountered] an overly strict confessor'.[25] Thus could a relevant assessment of piety and religious practice be appropriately incorporated into the case history, though not always smoothly, and not always unchallenged.[26]

From a psychiatric perspective – and even more that of liberal critics of Catholicism – the Redemptorist popular missions represented a genuine problem, especially for very pious and conscientious Tyroleans.[27] In 1845 Sebastian Ruf, the house chaplain at Hall, dryly informed his Bavarian friend and travel writer Ludwig Steub: 'Since the lay missions have delivered so many individuals to our asylum, the government saw fit to restrict [the missions] severely.'[28] And in 1846, the highly critical national liberal Matthias Koch reported on this same matter in his travel reportage on the sermons of the Tyrolean lay missions, who – in order to achieve their purpose – provoked strong 'emotional upset' and who presupposed

> that their listeners were obdurately serious sinners. If by some accident they were not, then they were rather conscientious or even scrupulous people. The disadvantageous effect of such emotionally upsetting sermonizing on these minds is to cause excruciating anxiety and even a degree of dangerous excitement. This actually happens not infrequently in Tyrol, and sometimes with lamentable consequences.[29]

24 The application of theological enlightenment in terms of sensible Christian religion as moral philosophy is outlined in Kaufmann, *Aufklärung, bürgerliche Selbsterfahrung und die 'Erfindung' der Psychiatrie*, 61.

25 Tschallener, *Beschreibung der k. k. Provinzial-Irren-Heilanstalt zu Hall in Tirol*, 67.

26 In the view of many contemporary physicians, and also some clergy, religious scruples were promoted by overly zealous confessors; but some physicians did raise tentative doubts in the medical records about this blanket attribution.

27 The order of Redemptorists was founded by Alphonsus Liguori. In 1749, the order was canonically approved by Pope Benedict XIV. In 1820, shortly after the death of Redemptorist and Viennese patron Klemens Maria Hofbauer, the order was also introduced into the Austrian states. In 1827, the first friars met at Innsbruck. From the 1840s, popular missions were established throughout the country.

28 Steub, *Sängerkrieg in Tirol*, 93.

29 Koch, *Reise in Tirol*, 186.

'Fire-and-brimstone sermons and advice in the confessional box' as well as reading 'excessively religious books' were regularly cited in the Hall patient files as triggers for religiously hued mental illness.[30] Another, equally frequent complaint was nonprofessional treatment by clergy. 'Now the relatives sought assistance everywhere, but rarely appropriately, until they reached a clergyman, who also failed to rid the body of the Devil', grumbled Tschallener.[31] Within the asylum, the chaplain-led religious practices of confession, communion, and attendance at mass represented key stages on the road to mental recovery. Masses in particular were ascribed a function akin to social therapy. Within the asylum walls, confession was used as a means of regulating the troubled relationship between 'true piety' and 'pathological exaggeration'. The idea was to allow patients to appeal to God's mercy while at the same time diluting the fear of eternal damnation, which Tschallener blamed on harsh and fanatical surroundings. In her gender-specific investigation of confessions in the nineteenth century, Edith Saurer notes that during this time, theology generally attached to confession a new, therapeutic value: to promote 'peace of mind'.[32] Thus, moderate pastoral models were largely consistent with the concept of psycho-moral treatment in contemporary insane asylums, a state of affairs confirmed by Herman Westerink in conjunction with French psychiatry around 1800.[33] To wit: physicians and clergy were broadly agreed on the view that fanatically overheated and exaggerated religiosity made people 'sick'. As a therapeutic tool, both groups had access only to the 'normally very limited religious knowledge of the common people' and their 'equally limited grasp of God and his characteristics'[34] gleaned from the asylum clergy at Hall, through religious instruction given separately for both sexes, in German and Italian. Even the medical director considered himself up to the task of religious instruction. Tschallener reported the treatment of a young male patient as follows:

> I now simply took this person to my room and offered him all the words and comfort [I could think of] to relieve him of his delusion of inevitable, eternal damnation, which in fact was so effective that N. N. requested confession, which was also granted him. However, this confession did not go as hoped. N. told me a few days later, when on his request I again took him to my room, that he had not been entirely honest with the chaplain. A renewed and most forbearing instruction and productive solace brought the patient to a second confession and recovery. [Then] communion, and from this time forward he showed the most

30 Tschallener, *Beschreibung der k. k. Provinzial-Irren-Heilanstalt zu Hall in Tirol*, 162-163.
31 Ibid., 147.
32 Saurer, 'Frauen und Priester'.
33 Westerink, 'Demonic Possession', 336.
34 Tschallener, *Beschreibung der k. k. Provinzial-Irren-Heilanstalt zu Hall in Tirol*, 164.

> unmistakable improvement; N. N. regained his peace of mind, began to discover new pluck and zest for life, and up to the end of May conducted himself to our greatest satisfaction.[35]

In one of the earliest manuals for German institutional psychiatry, Johann Christian Reil's *Rhapsodieen über die Anwendung der psychischen Kurmethode auf Geisteszerrüttungen* (1803) the author called for another type of staff for the 'healing institution' as opposed to a custodial institution, namely, 'specifically trained physicians, clerics, and philosophers', and more: 'Curing the insane requires proper allocation [of staff], great effort, and also a quiet struggle with the powers that be.'[36] On the basis of this characterization, the options for assisting and the positions of the asylum clergy were already embedded in just such a power play from the very beginning of institutional psychiatry; and yet in subsequent years they were increasingly the subject of contemporary controversies within the small group of German-speaking psychiatrists. Four decades after Reil, Hall's director Johann Tschallener represented a clear idea of the right balance of power and correspondingly appropriate teamwork between medicine and pastoral care within the asylum. First, collaboration with the asylum chaplain should strive to achieve the official goal of the hospital (cure), and to promote and represent this goal to the world outside. Second, Tschallener envisioned a detailed plan for religious instruction, tailored to sex and linguistic affiliation. Among other things, the chaplain was to say mass twice a week and to lead the rosary daily. In addition, the chaplain was to act as a sort of moral authority in the asylum and, together with the physicians, embody the humanitarian principles of modern care for the insane – not least with an eye to the wardens, who were generally described as crude and ignorant.[37] The main tasks of the Catholic house chaplain also included hearing confessions, the purpose of which, according to Tschallener, was 'to seek and to diligently exploit the expert opinion of the director and medical superintendent'.[38] In his descriptions of the asylum as well as in his therapeutic approach, Tschallener leaned on Johann Christian August Heinroth's *Textbook of Disturbances of Mental Life; or, Disturbances of the Soul and Their Treatments.* For Heinroth, as for Reil, philosophers were hardly suited as staff for a healing institution 'because their activity is confined to the writing desk',[39] and the cleric should only go to the aid of physicians in the case of those few patients who showed themselves to be exceptionally receptive to spiritual influence.

35 Tschallener, *Beschreibung der k. k. Provinzial-Irren-Heilanstalt zu Hall in Tirol*, 182.
36 Reil, *Rhapsodieen über die Anwendung der psychischen Kurmethode*, 20-21.
37 See Vanja, 'Madhouses, Children's Wards, and Clinics', 124.
38 Tschallener, *Beschreibung der k. k. Provinzial-Irren-Heilanstalt zu Hall in Tirol*, 40.
39 Heinroth, *Lehrbuch der Störungen des Seelenlebens*, 44-45. The citation here is from the English translation: Id., *Textbook of Disturbances of Mental Life*, 26.

> The clerics, as the recognized shepherds of the soul, are just as unfit for the tasks, owing to their point of view and the training and direction they have received. For their field of activity is the moral nature of man for as long as it exists and not after it has died or at least temporarily disappeared. Their business, their profession, is thus concerned with a sphere which is quite different from the one with which the doctor of the soul must be familiar.[40]

To summarize: within the newly structured and secularized landscape of medical care, the competence of physicians and clerics to treat mental illness was, on the one hand, sometimes contentious. On the other hand, the relationship between religion and medical and psychiatric approaches to pathologically religious phenomena was far more complex than the unfolding historical accounts of success and professionalization in psychiatry during the period under study both then and to date would lead one to suspect. As an example of the discourse around demonic possession, Herman Westerink convincingly cites a contemporary nineteenth-century myth, according to which 'modern treatment of mental illness began with an anticlerical victory over [...] religion's ignorance of madness'.[41] During the 1800s, the house chaplains at Hall accentuated their ambivalent position in the force field of the modern asylum in different ways – based on their individual professional strategies and divergent ideological interests.[42] Without delving more into detail regarding the scope for treatment and decision making of this group, what follows will nonetheless shed light on exemplary conflicts, rivalries, and collaborations based on patient files that, in my opinion, also have something to do with the fact that common knowledge in medicine and religion, and its interpretation, always also includes uncertain knowledge.

Uncertain knowledge: the challenge of therapeutic practice

The medical record of Josepha S* indicates that both contemporary medical cures and religious solace played a role in therapy. In her sad, doubtful state of mind, the patient herself asked 'whether the alleged influence of the Evil Enemy within her' might respond to 'spiritual methods and benedictions', as noted for example in March 1844. Her wishes in this matter were respected by the asylum. However, in May 1844 it was further noted that the spiritual help 'was also of no avail'. In June, medical superintendent Johann Tschallener recorded that, in accordance with the chaplain, the patient was prohibited religious instruction following repeated instances of 'frighteningly violent

40 Ibid.
41 Westerink, 'Demonic Possession', 339.
42 Heidegger, 'Seelsorge in der frühen Anstaltspsychiatrie'.

attacks'. From July 1844, Josepha S* refused all medicines and desired help only from the clergy. In September 1844 it was again noted that the patient believed that 'only benediction and prayer would help, if that is still possible'. The reaction, in the words of the deputy physician, was that in the treatment of Josepha S*, 'everything possible' had been tried:

> As our Rev[erend] Chaplain no longer seemed to suffice, we allowed a Franciscan priest to come to her, but nothing worked. Indeed, the more her condition deteriorated, the more this respect of her wishes seemed to encourage her delusion; she suffers greatly, is very emaciated, and her appearance is getting worse and worse, ...[she] feels as if something alive (the Devil) is sending a lightning bolt through her body; the merest thought of her condition, often the glimpse of an unfamiliar cleric, or some other slight event, is enough to provoke in her the most violent convulsions.

The further course of therapy in the case of Josepha S* showed little change. In September 1844 she was again forbidden to go to church, on a trial basis, to see 'what effect that might have on her'; 'but as she now refused to follow any orders, the result was disappointing'. Three months later, in December 1844, she persisted in her delusion

> that the Evil One was working his mischief on her; she believed that help was to be found only with the clergy, although that had already been tried; at her own request the Rev[erend] Dean had several times been summoned, resulting in a few hours of relative calm; but then even on the same day it was the same old story: the usual convulsions, especially of the head, and the extremities, and then anew pleas for us to allow this or that cleric to come, or to write to the bishop.

Finally, in February 1845, the patient was sent back home 'uncured', after (according to the final, succinct entry in the record) her condition not only failed to improve during her stay in the asylum 'but even worsened'.[43] Thus hardly a success story. The monthly entries in Josepha S*'s file describe routine therapy in brief and blunt terms, that is, outside of a macro-historical interpretive context and subject to the professional positioning of the challenging processes of modernization, medicalization, and secularization. The application of appropriate (from a medical perspective) psycho-pedagogical and pharmacological treatment methods, compatible with secular concepts of religious pathology, posed a daily challenge from the vantage of experienced suffer-

43 HA LKH, Krankenakten Frauen 1845, Josepha S* I/204, Irrenprotokolle.

ing. In addition, there were moments of uncertainty that basically escaped the considerations of history of psychiatry. At issue was namely day-to-day and case-by-case practical medical knowledge, or rather the practical relevance of indirect claims to medical knowledge. And although it was extremely unlikely that Hall patient Josepha S* was in fact be possessed by the devil, a degree of significance had to be accorded her subjective knowledge in this practical dimension such that it forced appreciable concessions in her treatment. But the records cited here left little space for scholarly references, lengthy interpretations, or moralizing discussion. Rather, they effectively communicated the increasing disinterest of physicians as the asylum stay wore on. The longer and more routine the presence of a patient in the asylum, the more laconic and circumspect the corresponding record of practical medical knowledge.[44]

Since the 1980s the social history of medicine has jockeyed for greater recognition of the patient's perspective. Medical records were discovered and explored as polyphonic sources, inasmuch as they offered access to the suffering of patients. More recently, calls have been made for more attention to the 'insights' of staff[45] – physicians as well as nurses and other actors within the psychiatric arena. Initially, interest focused on strategic staging of the phases of professionalization and the history of science agenda. Now, the focus has turned to therapeutic intentions. However, as a result, the question also arises how to represent uncertainties in diagnosis and treatment, questions of fear, loyalty conflicts, and feelings of responsibility that, during the period under study, were increasingly recognized as the social sequelae of mental suffering. I assert that it is precisely interpretive leeway in the range of signs and symptoms requiring interpretation that generates uncertain knowledge and the unending search for evidence. The visible convulsions of Josepha S*, which physicians interpreted as hysteria, convinced them that they were dealing with an illness for which appropriate medical terminology existed. In October 1843, when Josepha S* was no longer willing to tell the doctors about her 'being possessed by the Devil', as far as they were concerned, her madness was 'only too obvious' based on her actions, 'signs of the cross, prayers, incantations'.[46] If the visibility of medically interpreted and functionalized signs amounts to medical knowledge, then conversely the non-visibility of a devil or demon amounts to uncertainty. At the time, neither the affected persons, the relatives, nor even the physicians could entirely rule out the devil's existence or direct influence, not to mention a supernatural origin of physical signs. Pastoral and contemporary medicine found in this uncertainty common ground regarding both sin and disease, whereby, as Waltraud Pulz writes, 'Overlaps between medical and religious discourse' were even the rule and produced

44 Heidegger, 'Körper – Seele – Leid', 141.
45 See, for example, Vanja, 'Das Irrenhaus als Totale Institution?', 128.
46 HA LKH, Krankenakten Frauen 1845, Josepha S* I/204, Irrenprotokolle.

'complex structures'.[47] In this complex constellation, treatment of religious melancholics and lunatics involved a set of simultaneous interventions that were not necessarily in competition with each other. This was also the case with 29-year-old Anna G*, a farmer's daughter, who likewise received a diagnosis of 'religious melancholy in a hysterical individual' and died in the Hall asylum of exhaustion in 1837. Until the very last she was tormented by visions in which she saw the sky as black and the moon blood-red, and perceived omens in the sky that told her she was damned. The nights brought no peace because 'the Evil One' plagued her. Her relatives treated the suicidal Anna G* 'lovingly' and 'observed [her] closely'; 'therapy' consisted of bloodletting and 'sedatives' as well as (obviously) 'all spiritual means required'.[48] According to the entries in her patient file, Anna G* suffered from visibly hysterical convulsions and invisible symptoms of spiritual disturbance and madness; in addition to her hallucinations, 'she had committed all manner of sins and thus had no hope of bliss'. Anna's treatment provided for walks outside the asylum walls, including to a clergyman 'whom she trusted'; within the walls she occupied herself with reading from her childhood library, from which, however, her prayer books had 'quietly been removed' as a precaution. Unfortunately, after the position of asylum chaplain was vacated in July 1836, no one else was able to 'gain her trust'. To this entry by the assisting physician, asylum director Johann Tschallener added the lament: 'It is to be regretted that she is already feeling the absence of religious psychological aid; may this shameful inconvenience be remedied!'[49]

The patient-oriented focus in the treatment of Josepha S* and Anna G* shows that, contrary to the contemporary view of the inconvenience if not harmfulness of such influences, experiments in pastoral treatment in the form of 'religious psychological aid' were not excluded even in the treatment of religious melancholy or religious insanity. More decisive was the question of who should be allowed how much of this treatment, and who was entitled to make an appropriate diagnosis and to decide the quality and quantity of pastoral care. In this psychiatric context, and during the period under study, physicians clearly had claims to legitimate knowledge over clergy and especially over afflicted patients as well as exclusive competence to make such common diagnoses as 'lunacy' or 'melancholy in a hysterical individual' when a patient imagined him- or herself to be possessed by the devil or forever lost and damned. In this field of activity, exorcism and benedictions were clearly associated with ineffectiveness, and the entries in the patient files reflect relevant disputes relating to pastoral intervention vis-à-vis the troubled soul. But though the asylum's treatment program was focused on curing madness,

47 Pulz, 'Krank versus gesund?', 83.
48 HA LKH, Krankenakten Frauen 1837, Anna G* I/88, Irrengeschichte.
49 Ibid., Irrenprotokolle.

and not expelling devils or demons from the body, from the perspective of therapeutic practice, the border between legitimate medical knowledge and the experiential knowledge of patients was not so sharply drawn. In fact, it appears as if the central predicament in the application of legitimate and authorized knowledge was the issue of compromise. The reasons were obvious: on the one hand, the insane asylum was not isolated from society, or from the contemporary ideological and political camps and intensified forms of piety unfolding within it. On the other hand, within the asylum, religious practitioners were structuring space and time in the form of the daily rosary recitation, twice-weekly masses, and the observance of holidays and religiously prescribed fasts. In the asylum, the medical treatment program and the practice of Catholic piety to some extent followed the same rhythm.[50] In the context of individual moral recovery, therapeutic practice also strove to take into account the emotional (religious) needs of patients or even a negative and punitive approach, such as withholding certain books or forbidding attendance at mass. Attempts were made again and again to somehow secure access to a 'diseased' mind and 'by any means', which also included routinely making compromises, such as permitting cooperation with non-asylum clergy outside the institution. This view is supported empirically by detailed analysis of historical patient files. The progress reports recorded by various physicians, which reveal sometimes diverging evaluations and suggestions, are particularly instructive. Occasionally, the debate over pathological forms of religiosity and the proper degree of healthy piety turned quite controversial, with the asylum clergy not necessarily representing the position of the 'sacred'.

All the more so because, from the perspective of pastoral care and pastoral psychiatry, which was developing in parallel with mainstream psychiatry, a reasonable and 'mature' religiosity and a 'beautiful religious world view' that was counter to a pathological and unbending religiosity and for the most part – without questioning the existence of the devil – was brought into play to combat possible cases of possession initially using earthly means.[51] Indeed, until very recently, according to the pastoral medical system it was possible that 'a demonic influence was at work in addition to natural factors or was secondarily grafted onto them'. As Albert Niedermeyer wrote in the 1950s, some 'manifestations of psychopathology and hysteria' represented 'fertile ground for demonic influence', whereby 'individual factors [could be teased apart] only with great difficulty'. Moreover, it was possible to imagine 'an increasing level of demonic influence... [that] may be slight at the beginning and

50 On piety as the rhythmic impulse of daily life, see De Giorgio, 'Die Gläubige', 123.

51 For a standard reference on the history of pastoral medicine, see Pompey, *Die Bedeutung der Medizin*. On the determinative positioning of special pastoral medicine with reference to canonical law, see Niedermeyer, *Handbuch der speziellen Pastoralmedizin*, in particular, the chapter on super- and preternatural phenomena.

then gradually take on weight, especially when the patient shows no resistance and entertains thoughts of obsession'.[52] Faced with this threat to salvation and peace of mind, spiritual healing assumed responsibility not only for the hereafter but also the here and now. Consequently, the clergy lay claim to therapeutic skills within the realm of psychiatry, and even medical knowledge. Sebastian Ruf (1802-1877), the house chaplain at Hall from 1837 to 1872, mentioned above, one of many Tyrolean clerics who as a young man could not afford a medical education in faraway Vienna, actively participated in the cause of modern psychiatry in Tyrol.[53] Ruf advocated a secular understanding of religion as a form of treatment. In a letter to his friend Ludwig Steub, Ruf described this personally motivated and morally and philosophically oriented therapeutic approach in this way:

> I have as little trust in my convictions as I do in my faith. Our conundrum can only be resolved in the hereafter, if such a thing exists. Kant and Fichte are of little use in reaching my lunatics. But a beautiful passage from the Bible and the promise of a better world lifts them up. When I observe the beneficial effect, I am sometimes moved to believe it myself.[54]

Like-minded liberal friends of Ruf assumed him to be an atheist in priest's clothing who had long finished with Catholicism. Following the March revolution, he also appeared as an author of socio-political newspaper articles in which, among other things, he discussed the phenomenon of mental illness in historical context. The uncertain knowledge in the face of therapeutic challenges in the asylum was reflected at yet another level: an experience of general uncertainty in one of the transitional periods experienced as such by contemporaries, which was characterized among other things by a revitalization of intensely pious practices. In this article I can only begin to touch on how these two dimensions of uncertain knowledge are related. Classifying the many different voices in the patient files in the broader context of the history of thought and religion requires a work of much greater scope.

The medical discourse on religious pathologies took place – or so I would maintain – in a historical context experienced by contemporaries like Ruf as a time 'suspended between good and evil':[55] Tyrol was repeatedly described as backward and conservative; its society was dominated by the Catholic Church, whose reactionary political and clerical decision makers embraced religious unity in the German-speaking part of the country and successfully

52 Niedermeyer, *Handbuch der speziellen Pastoralmedizin*, 431.
53 Lentner, *Sebastian Ruf*.
54 Steub, *Sängerkrieg in Tirol*, 83.
55 Ruf, 'Gymnastische Uebung'.

drove dissenters out of the Ziller valley in 1837. In this spatial and temporal context, the question of the competence to treat mental illnesses also acquired a philosophical and political dimension. There was, for example, the famous (and for the Hall physicians, infamous) pre-March case of the Tyrolean pastor Simon Alois Maaß, whose treatment of 'possessed' and 'melancholic' patients was repeatedly attested to and criticized in the Hall patient files. Maaß worked from 1805 to 1846 as a pastor in Fließ, a small mountain village in the Upper Inn valley in Tyrol, as a sort of emergency helper – especially as confessor and exorcist – when all other means and actors fell short. An avowed conservative during the transitional period, Maaß was naturally also a strong opponent of smallpox vaccination. His view was that it enabled the mixing of humans and animals, which in turn would increase offenses against the rule of chastity; in his rectory he treated a long line of moody women and suicidal junior priests and collaborators who were sent by church officials to be billeted with him. Maaß was alleged to have substantial naturopathic knowledge and to have worked with a pharmacist and surgeon on the best of terms; indeed, the latter was said to have prospered from his association with the pastor. In 1837 the district office charged Maaß with the unauthorized practice of medical arts and 'serious infringement of the law'. But for healing the 'afflicted' and 'melancholy' as part of so-called 'private exorcism', the pastor had the approval of the archbishop. For this purpose, in addition to the sacramentals, he used sacred crosses, medals, rosaries, herbs, and oils. On the strength of a supreme decree dating back to 1755, according to which no priest was allowed to carry out exorcisms without state approval, Maaß was said to have been confronted by the government for his exorcisms. According to his biographer, the pastor's response (which, unfortunately, cannot be corroborated) was to say: 'I did not realize that the Devil was a matter for government.'[56]

The psychiatric history of Maria P*, a maidservant from Hall, recounts the patient's lengthy stay with pastor Maaß. Previously, soon after experiencing hallucinations in which she heard nagging voices, the young woman's relatives entrusted her to the care of a Franciscan priest, because her parents suspected that 'the <u>devil</u> [emphasis in the original] wishe[d] to play his fateful game with this young girl'. The case history goes on to name a number of other actors and hospitals. However, Maria P* turns out not simply to have been a passive sufferer who was treated here and there and sent hither and yon – and it is in this sense that her history serves to complement my thesis – but rather also as an individual with a will of her own:

> The Rev[erend] Father told her that she had to transform herself from the soles of her feet up; admonished her to make thrice-weekly confessions in addition to other exercises in devotion; and ultimately granted

56 Bader, *Der alte Fließer Pfarrer*, 252.

> her a blanket forgiveness. But this asceticism was little to the patient's liking, and consequently both patient and spiritual healer tired of each other. Soon her parents sent her to another priest in the area, who gave her his benediction 9 days in a row... Finally, she was handed over to the Rev[erend] Dean ['Dekan'], who barely achieved any better success through appropriate religious influence.[57]

Now the relatives again sought the help of a doctor, whom the young woman saw regularly for two months and who advised the parents to try to have their mad daughter admitted to the insane asylum. But Maria P* resisted, deciding instead to leave her hometown and to go work in various places in Tyrol and Switzerland as a maidservant

> in the hope of finally escaping her alleged pursuers. But neither the great distance from home nor the psychic treatment of the late Pastor in Fließ did much to alleviate her dismal mental state. Because the aforementioned Pastor assured the unhappy girl that both the apparitions and the unsettling voices were partly the work of the Devil and partly the work of bad, immoral louts and strumpets, and that she was herself perfectly healthy in body, she henceforth anxiously avoided the society of young people; but she persisted in her claims of hallucinations. Now, after nearly 2 years, the afflicted girl finally decided of her own accord to seek her last refuge in the [Hall] insane asylum, which she had previously fearfully avoided.[58]

In the progress reports attached to the file, the wilfulness of the patient is repeatedly emphasized, including in the entries made by Hall house chaplain Sebastian Ruf. In January 1849, Ruf noted: 'P. is pious, but after her own manner. She is beset by struggles with lewd spirits. Incidentally, she attends church and instruction.' In February 1849, he wrote: 'P. seeks help from the priest in her fight against temptations and promptings. Requests benediction. Goes to church and instruction', and in May 1849: 'P. can hardly be swayed in religious matters; here, too, she goes her own way and attends instruction or not depending on her mood.'[59]

57 HA LKH, Krankenakten Frauen 1849, Maria P* I/268, Krankengeschichte.
58 Ibid.
59 Ibid., Irrenprotokolle.

Conclusion

The strong element of individuality that is expressed in the entries on Maria P* provokes a few concluding thoughts. A micro-historical research program rooted in the 'little narratives' contained in the patient files with unexpected, individual snapshots, experiences, and biographical fragments, is also and always critically concerned with the so-called 'grand narratives' of secularization, modernization, professionalization, and medicalization. It focuses on rifts that reveal a shift in perspective in these grand narratives. In modern Western societies, for example, according to a classical and increasingly obsolete theory of modernization, the different areas of social life grew apart. Consequently, secularization is seen as a process in which religious ideas, practices, and organizations increasingly forfeited their overall social influence and gradually lost their legitimacy vis-à-vis scientific knowledge. However, empirical studies of historical religious practices and experiences of devotion in the nineteenth and twentieth centuries have revised this idea of secularization and, with it, the classical thesis of disenchantment with the world (Max Weber). Furthermore, it can now be shown that religion was actively involved in the cultural modernity project.[60]

Within the psychiatric healing institution of the first half of the nineteenth century – which positioned itself contemporarily as a modernity project in a transitional period and wished to be perceived as such – the coexistence of a secular understanding of psychiatric illness and health, and a theological concept of pastoral care and salvation, can now be demonstrated through the patient files. This, to my mind, conveys the overriding impression that with respect to the melancholic and religiously insane patients admitted to the asylum, and in view of the related therapeutic challenges and the social backgrounds of such patients (mostly from the lower levels of society), no monopoly on secularly determined truth could be enforced. Both inside the asylum and outside its walls, pastoral and medical custody and dependency relationships existed side by side. Although pastoral and psychiatric actors were in competition with one another, just as often they cooperated in light of common concern for afflicted souls.[61]

Even the devil, it seems, refused to be driven from the asylum. At the most, he was pushed to the periphery from time to time through the collective daily efforts of the medical and spiritual personnel to rid the body and mind of 'demonic possession'.[62] The entries in the monthly progress reports suggest that medical treatment focused less on the repeatedly observed and

60 See Cox, 'Secularization and Other Master Narratives of Religion'; Ziemann, 'Säkularisierung, Konfessionalisierung, Organisationsbildung'; Borutta, 'Genealogie der Säkularisierungstheorie'.

61 See Heidegger, 'Handlungsräume und Positionen von Anstaltsgeistlichen', 274.

62 See Schön, *Mittheilungen aus dem Leben Geistesgestörter*, 183.

recorded physical signs interpreted as hysterical convulsions. In other words, the prescribed sedatives and soothing applications to the body served not to obliterate the signs but rather to reach the mind by treating the body. Physical signs were in fact of key significance in ascertaining truth for diagnostic practices. But their relevance appears to have declined in the everyday setting of therapeutic practice.[63]

The fundamental question is whether a secularized, cure- and future-oriented approach to the problem of religious pathologies under medical and pastoral care could be achieved in the face of the prevailing emphasis on the hereafter. This is, after all, what gives modern medical facilities their legitimacy. For sure, a focus on healing in this world was part of the new asylum program and had already long been part of medical identity. Yet given the many cases in the Tyrolean asylum patient files documenting ambiguous, fantasy-rich obsession, and religious interpretations of meaning, suffering, and fear of hell, it may be assumed that the asylum, like other institutions, was also a place where the process of secularization failed to be fully realized because transcendent healing never lost its importance.

63 Christina Vanja describes this aptly: 'When medical treatment was unsuccessful, people gave up on healing and simply awaited death. At that point, the individual's relationship with God needed to be sorted out.' Vanja, 'Madhouses, Children's Wards, and Clinics', 125.

GUSTAVE BOISSARIE, JEAN-MARTIN CHARCOT AND SIGMUND FREUD

THREE DOCTORS' RESPONSES TO SOME UNUSUAL BODILY PHENOMENA: CONVERGENCES AND DIVERGENCES (IN THE LATE NINETEENTH AND EARLY TWENTIETH CENTURIES)

NICOLE EDELMAN

In the late nineteenth and early twentieth centuries, the doctors Gustave Boissarie (1836-1917), director of the Lourdes Medical Bureau (Bureau des Constatations médicales), Jean-Martin Charcot (1825-1893) at La Salpêtrière Hospital in Paris and Sigmund Freud (1856-1939) at his practice in Vienna interpreted a number of similar physical phenomena such as convulsions, visions and paralysis. They wrote extensively on the subject, and each man's writings have been analysed by historians. However, comparisons between them have invariably been between pairs: either Boissarie and Charcot or, more commonly, Freud and Charcot. Yet their interpretations led all three to ask questions about belief and the role it played in the expression and form of these phenomena. They also considered their origins. How should the aetiology of these tangible signs be understood? Were they due to purely neurological dysfunctions or to a psychological malaise? Such questions were especially urgent during a fin de siècle period in which controversy between science and religion was rife.

The places where these phenomena were observed were the Catholic countries of France and Austria, at the great hospital of La Salpêtrière in Paris and at certain pilgrimage sites: Mariazell in Austria and the prestigious Lourdes. France played a particular role in this field, with important debates taking place there in the final decade of the nineteenth century and the first few of the twentieth. Although most of these phenomena were not new, having featured in descriptions of hysteria or possession for centuries, during these decades they acquired an exceptional character through the great violence of their form, the interest aroused by media coverage of them and the fierceness of the controversies they inspired. The major hysterical seizures of La Salpêtrière that Charcot demonstrated in the amphitheatre of his hospital recalled the days of demonic possession. They gave rise to controversy among doctors, some of whom also levelled accusations against the Catholic authorities, especially Désiré-Magloire Bourneville, a close associate of Charcot, who claimed that they had burnt sick people on the grounds that they were demonic, possessed or practitioners of witchcraft.[1] Some of these hysterics who were hospitalized at La Salpêtrière were sent by Charcot to Lourdes, where a number of healings duly took place. And although Catholic doctors at the shrine attributed some of these healings to miracles, Charcot strongly disagreed. Since the apparitions of Mary experienced by Bernadette Soubirous in 1858 and recognized by the Catholic church authorities in 1862[2], Lourdes had become an internationally renowned place of pilgrimage and its miracles were examined before being validated or rejected by a Medical Bureau that was established in 1883 and directed by Dr Gustave Boissarie[3] from 1892 until his death.[4] The Catholic doctors thus found themselves up against the Parisian neurologist Jean-Martin Charcot, who was likewise a figure of international renown. The hysteria specialist argued that these physical phenomena were related to hysteria and that the Lourdes healings had non-miraculous causes. The debate was all the fiercer as the French government of the Third Republic was at odds with the Catholic authorities, which in general were deeply hostile to the new regime with its secular aspirations. After the publication in 1893 of *La foi qui guérit* (an article originally written in English as *The Faith Cure*) by Jean-Martin Charcot and then of Émile Zola's novel *Lourdes* in 1894, which was hugely successful (as well as being blacklisted), the debate went international. Although Freud was not directly involved, he is known to have had close ties with Charcot, having worked alongside him in Paris for a few months in 1885-86. He was very familiar with his work, and Charcot's observation of hysterics is also known to have been essential to Freud's development of psychoanalysis. Moreover, his psychoanalytical medical approach soon led him to question the place of religion both in human society and in the lives of individuals, especially as he himself had encountered strong anti-Semitism in Catholic Austria.[5] He was also acquainted with anti-Semitism in France, not only through the Dreyfus Affair and the role of Zola, whom he admired and whose work he rated highly, but also through the anti-Semitic attacks suffered

1 Regnard and Bourneville, *L'iconographie de la Salpêtrière*.

2 Harris, *Lourdes*.

3 Boissarie, *Lourdes, histoire médicale*; Id., *Lourdes depuis 1858*; Id., *Les grandes guérisons de Lourdes* and articles in *Annales de Notre Dame de Lourdes*.

4 Guise-Castelnuovo, 'Le docteur Boissarie et les "guéris" de Lourdes'.

5 *The Future of an Illusion* and *Compulsive Actions and Religious Exercises* were published in 1927 and 1907.

by the doctor Hippolyte Bernheim with whom he stayed in 1889 and certain of whose works on suggestion and hypnotism he translated.[6] The text *Une névrose démoniaque au XVII*[e] *siècle* (*Eine Teufelneurose im Siebzehnten Jahrhundert / A Neurosis of Demoniacal Possession in the Seventeenth Century*), published in 1923, which describes a man afflicted by convulsions, visions, and paralysis which lead him to make a pilgrimage to Mariazell, therefore seems to me to serve as a counterpoint to the writings of Boissarie and Charcot, especially as Charcot also analysed phenomena from the past in two of his publications: *La foi qui guérit* (*The Faith Cure*) and *Les démoniaques dans l'art* (*Demoniacs in Art*).

Charcot, Boissarie and Freud, like most doctors in Europe and North America at that time, were trained in clinical observation, and all three had had lengthy contact with the hospital world – in France in the case of the first two, and throughout Europe more generally in the case of Freud. They were all doctors whose reputation extended well beyond France or Austria. There were thus plenty of similarities between them, and all three had learned to identify the signs of an illness through observation performed during the physical and mental examination of a patient, in order to diagnose in accordance with a nosological classification defined by their medical knowledge. They were able to contrast these observed signs, which were deemed to be objective, with symptoms that were open to interpretation, because they were a way for the patient to express an illness or malaise through his body. The patient could thus invent, imagine or transform what he thought he felt. In this way, the subjective world-view of each participant in the diagnosis became a relevant factor: that of the patient, and that of the doctor looking at the patient as an individual and hence capable of judging him by his beliefs. Boissarie, Charcot and Freud thus diverged in their interpretation of these exceptional, yet similar-looking physical phenomena. We will now observe and analyse these divergences through certain of the writings of these three doctors.

For Charcot, although the observed physical phenomena were exceptional, they were also ancient manifestations, 'since time immemorial', as he put it. While working at La Salpêtrière Hospital in the late 1870s, he came to believe that he had identified, beneath the apparent disorder of hysteria, a hidden order in the condition's attacks. He emphasized the regularity of their structure, referring to four phases which, he claimed, succeeded one another in an attack of hysteria: 1) epileptoid fits; 2) contortions and grand movements; 3) passionate attitudes; 4) delirium; each of these phases had its own somatic characteristics. In his book written with Paul Richer, *Les démoniaques dans l'art*, he re-examined a vast range of drawings, engravings and paintings from the past and found all the signs of the great 'hysterical neurosis', as he defined

6 He knew the works of Zola, whom he admired. In 1906, he cited *Fecundity* as one of the ten best books. He also had at least two books on Zola's life in his library in London.

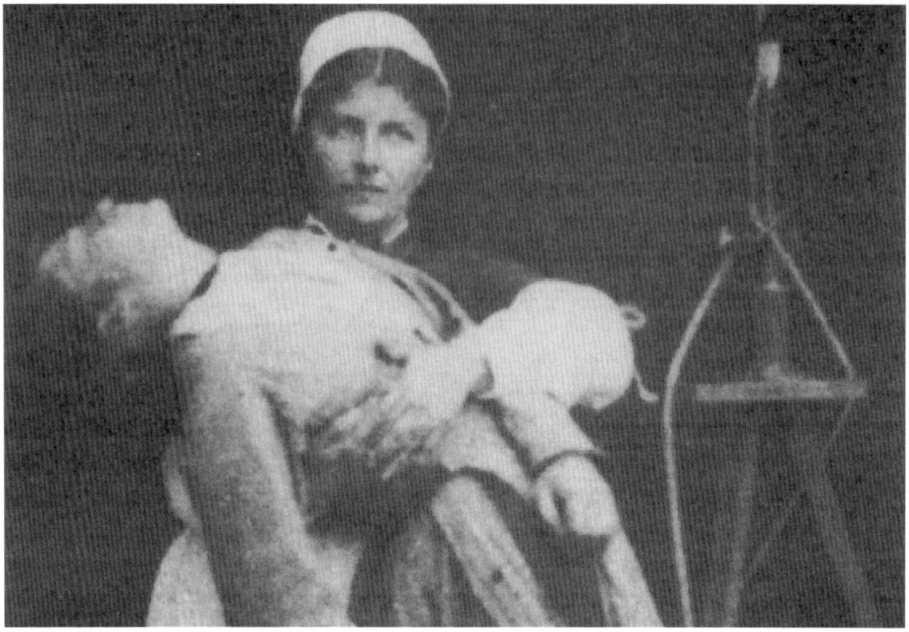

'Léthargie, résultant de la suppression brusque de la lumière'.
[*Paul Regnard and Désiré-Magloire Bourneville.* Iconographie photographique de la Salpêtrière (service de M. Charcot). *Vol. 3, picture 8. Paris, 1880*]

it in the light of his knowledge. Rather than looking for distinctive or original traits in these works from previous centuries, he identified that which was analogous and similar only, projecting onto these representations contemporary traits he had identified in his patients, 'his' hysterics: auras, spasms, convulsions, paralyses and so on.[7] When he did not find the expected traits, for example in the 'Possessed boy' by Raphael (1520) in *The Transfiguration*, he claimed that 'such a master must have falsified and changed nature deliberately'.[8] Likewise, when on the eve of his death, in late 1892, he described certain atypical signs, namely ulcers and tumours, in his final publication, *La foi qui guérit* (*The Faith Cure*)[9], rather than treating them as symptoms of new diseases he related them to hysteria.[10] Just as he had demonstrated the similarity between the hysterics he was treating at La Salpêtrière and those depicted in old paintings, engravings or drawings, he now demonstrated the similarities between the different shrines which, in his view, were the decisive cause of miraculous healings.

7 Charcot and Richer, *Les démoniaques dans l'art*, followed by Charcot's *La foi qui guérit*, XXI.
8 Ibid., 31.
9 Charcot, 'La foi qui guérit', *Revue hebdomadaire*, 1892.
10 Id., *La foi qui guérit*, published in *Les démoniaques dans l'art*, 113.

What is especially interesting to study from the point of view of the determinism of the miracle is the shrine itself. And this determinism becomes striking when one observes that all shrines are alike, all are cast in the same mould. They have remained the same from the remotest periods of history to the present, copying each other, so to speak. For it is clear that through the ages, among the most diverse civilisations, amid the seemingly most dissimilar religions, the conditions of the miracle have remained the same, its evolutionary laws being immutable.[11]

Although Charcot never refers to Lourdes in this article, talking about the Asclepeion in Athens instead, his readers inevitably think of Lourdes. He concludes that: 'The implementation of faith healing, therefore, since time immemorial, in all latitudes, among pagans, Christians and Muslims, has had the same character. The shrines and propitiatory practices are similar. Only the statues of the healing god differ, but the human spirit, always the same in its main manifestations, prays at them all without differentiation.'[12]

Hysteria had thus produced similar phenomena for centuries, since as far as Charcot was concerned, its aetiology was purely neurological: it was due to a dynamic lesion *sine materia* of the brain that was as yet invisible, but that doctors would one day discover.[13] This dynamic lesion would appear and then disappear, and explained patients' nervous disorders and suffering. It could be caused by a nervous shock of the emotional type, which had a painful effect on the brain. Charcot therefore thought that a second psychological shock – caused by powerful self-suggestion, in a place charged with beliefs, such as a shrine – could bring about the remission and cure of the disease. He thus attributed a decisive role to self-suggestion (excluding hypnotism) in this type of healing.[14] Patients who were susceptible to healing therefore had to believe that they could be healed, and the mental state of hysterics was conducive to the development of such *faith* because they were highly suggestible. If the hysteric had certainty and absolute faith in her healing, the shock produced by the places of pilgrimage – a procession, a solemn blessing, immersion in the icy waters of a pool, an impressive ceremony – might be sufficient to cause all the symptoms of the disease to disappear.[15] For Charcot, the mechanism of such a cure was ultimately purely neurological in nature. In his view, the symptoms of hysterics expressed their genuine physical suffering, and therefore could be neither simulated nor invented. Such bodily phe-

11 Ibid., 114.
12 Ibid., 115.
13 Edelman, *Les métamorphoses de l'hystérique*.
14 Bernheim regarded hysteria as of psychological origin. It followed that 'hysterical fits, psycho-physiological reactions, phenomena of a purely dynamic nature, can in most cases be inhibited and eradicated by a psychological influence'. Conversely, he could provoke any succession of phases by the power of suggestion in an hysteric, including the four at La Salpêtrière.
15 Charcot, *La foi qui guérit*, published in *Les démoniaques dans l'art*, 122.

nomena did not express any intimate and personal malaise of a psychological nature.

The charismatic Charcot was confident of his science and of his international audience. As he saw it, the supernatural interpretation had dominated for centuries, but medical investigation was slowly pushing it back, and the inevitable onward march of modern scientific progress would ultimately prevail. 'The scientific order'[16] was triumphing, and faith healing was indeed a miracle – but a 'therapeutic miracle'[17] with nothing supernatural about it. He was certain that the rational and scientific interpretation would prevail one day, as ignorance receded and science made further inevitable advances. For Charcot, therefore, signs and symptoms overlapped.

For the Catholic doctors, and Gustave Boissarie in particular, the conclusions were more complex, and in many respects contradictory. Signs of hysteria and hysterics' symptoms were not always synonymous. They, too, were extremely sensitive to the pathological signs of sick people arriving in Lourdes. Baron Dunot de Saint-Maclou, resident physician at Lourdes from 1884 until his death in 1891, imparted a certain rigour to the procedures for examining the recipients of miracles, not least because of his familiarity with Charcot's work on hysteria and that of Hippolyte Bernheim in Nancy on hypnotism. He also established the Lourdes Medical Bureau, whose staff of doctors grew continuously and which was directed by Gustave Boissarie. The latter had been trained in Paris hospitals: he worked at La Charité Hospital, where he completed part of his internship with Pierre Briquet, a leading expert in hysteria before Charcot and the first to have claimed that hysteria was 'a neurosis of the brain'.[18] Boissarie therefore knew that hysteria could reproduce many of the functional disorders and signs of other diseases, and although he recognized that hysteria could be cured by an emotional shock (for example during a pilgrimage), he took the view firstly that the disease could not present signs such as tumours and ulcers, and secondly that certain cases of healings of hysterics did in fact constitute miracles. He made the Medical Bureau a very important place, and issued wide-ranging invitations to his colleagues to visit. Many doctors did so, often motivated by scientific curiosity. Charcot sent some of his hysterics there; healings of hysterics were said to be common in Lourdes, especially of those with paralysis, but Charcot himself never went there.

Given that the doctors of the Medical Bureau were devout Catholics, in their view, obviously, miracles really did happen: God, his saints or Mary could heal natural diseases. It was therefore essential for the clinical examination of recipients of miracles by the doctors at Lourdes to be beyond reproach. It was necessary to distinguish simulated illnesses from genuine ones, and of

16 Charcot, *La foi qui guérit*, published in *Les démoniaques dans l'art*, 111.

17 Ibid., 112.

18 'Neurosis' in the sense of 'a disease of the nerves' and not in the sense that Freud would give it.

course not to confuse natural and supernatural phenomena, saintliness and neurosis or divine ecstasy and pathological ecstasy. In these areas, doctors could rely both on the frameworks developed by the ecclesiastical authorities[19] and on the certainty that 'Catholic science' was, as had been openly proclaimed by scientists who were believers at the first International Scientific Congress of Catholics in Paris in 1888, a contradiction in terms. There could in fact only be one point of view, God could not be wrong, and there could be no contradiction between faith and science. These Catholic doctors could have absolute confidence in the future; their faith could not be contradicted by scientific progress. Only sincere faith on the part of the sick made miraculous cures possible, which presented no challenge to medical knowledge. Miracles fell within the category of the ineffable supernatural.

They therefore set about showing that the symptoms of miraculously cured hysterics were different in character from the symptoms of the hysterics in the hospitals. In 1890 and 1891, the *Annales de Lourdes* devoted a series of articles to 'Lourdes and Science' in which the question of the healing of nervous diseases was raised. Boissarie and his colleagues carefully examined the thesis of healing through religious suggestion and emotional shock. Their aim was to neutralize and reject the major objection raised by non-believing doctors, and by Charcot, that the overstimulation of the faith associated with the pilgrimage and the crowds, the self-suggestion of the procession to the Basilica of the Rosary, and the dips in the pools were enough to account for the healings. Although (like Charcot) they recognized that faith in healing could cause a temporary disappearance of the bodily signs of disease, they held that only a miracle could lead to a cure that was both immediate and, above all, free from relapse. This aspect of permanence was essential for the recognition of a miracle (as it still is today). From 1889, Dr Boissarie criticized Charcot's attempt to create experimental miracles, for example with the famous Etcheverry, one of the great hysterics treated by Charcot at La Salpêtrière. It was claimed that she had been instructed to recover from a nervous paralysis during a ceremony to mark the 'Month of Mary', and the paralysis had indeed disappeared at the desired moment.[20] Boissarie showed that the hysterics miraculously healed in Lourdes were different in character. They were simple and natural and their symptoms were real, not performed and dramatized, whereas the hospital illnesses were fabricated and they had been instructed what symptoms to display. They were artificial and fake, because the doctors had subjected them to numerous experiments in the induction of hypnosis (an accusation, incidentally, that was levelled at Bernheim, not Charcot). The Lourdes doctors thus argued that there were two types of hysterics: those on pilgrimage at Lourdes,

19 Debreyne (a medical doctor and religious brother of the order of La Grande Trappe), *Essai sur la théologie morale*, frequently reissued in the nineteenth century.

20 *Annales de Notre-Dame de Lourdes*, 1889, 56.

with their irreproachable morality and faith in God and Mary, and those at the large urban hospitals. The hysterical women (there were only a tiny number of men) who came on pilgrimage, impelled by a profound faith, were genuinely sick people, with the 'twofold burden of their illness and their duties', suffering women of 'truly exquisite moral qualities'.[21] In their own homes, 'one often observes the most outstanding qualities (...). Mind and heart do not bear the impression of their physical disorders. Even in the midst of these struggles and sufferings, their moral qualities appear to rise above the average level.'[22] By contrast, the picture presented of the hospital hysteric was damning. These hysterics were 'neurotic, unhinged, disturbed, physically and morally shattered by excessive and cruel experiments in hypnotism in which, after their freedom, their conscience and all sense of morality has been destroyed, they sometimes lose their reason.'[23] Boissarie added: 'I have seen these subjects, broken in and treated with scant respect (...), this herd of degraded creatures whose fits of laughter, profanities, erratic leaps and grimacing attitudes recalled the Fanatics of Saint Médard, and I reject any comparison between these desecrated hysterics, marked with the seal of the beast, and the sick at Lourdes, awaiting healing in all the beauty of human dignity, in prayer and serenity.'[24] Boissarie (like Charcot!) thus identified these physical phenomena of the women in the hospitals with the traits of possession in earlier centuries. They were said to be 'marked with the seal of the beast', they leapt and grimaced... Boissarie hinted that they might still be possessed by the devil... His moral judgment was implacable on the one group and highly complimentary on the other. In his view, signs and symptoms were indeed separate, and he seemed to think that the one group of women expressed a malaise caused by their doctors while the others exclusively expressed a genuine and proper physical condition. Finally, we may note the way in which Sigmund Freud analysed bodily phenomena equivalent to those of the hysterics. For him, the signs of hysteria were consistent with Charcot's analysis, but did not suggest a brain injury: in the context of the nascent science of psychoanalysis, they could be symptoms of representations that had been repressed, hidden and masked, because they were unacceptable, by the conscious part of the subject.

Freud examined these signs and symptoms by means of a kind of *clinical* examination of a case from the late seventeenth century that he discovered in a manuscript, part of which consisted of eight drawings and a journal written by the painter Christoph Haitzmann that was given to the religious of Mariazell during a pilgrimage. The analysis of these eight drawings and the journal, which Freud believed to be truthful, prompted the writing of

21 *Annales de Notre-Dame de Lourdes*, 1894, 310.
22 Boissarie, *Les grandes guérisons de Lourdes*, 456.
23 Ibid., X.XI.
24 Ibid., XI.

A Seventeenth-Century Demonological Neurosis.[25] Freud describes in this work the early symptoms of illness in the painter who, losing confidence in his art, afflicted by melancholy due to the death of his father and at a loss, claims to have yielded to the enticements of the devil, and to have signed a document in his own blood stating that he belonged body and soul to the devil.[26] Then, believing himself to be healed, the devil having given this first pact back to him, Haitzmann visits his sister, at whose house he enjoys a few months of remission.[27] However, new signs of disease appear, leading him to return to Mariazell[28], where serious attacks then occur: he has visions (not of the devil this time, but of Christ or of Mary), convulsive states accompanied with acute pains, and paralysis of the legs.[29] However, Freud does not stop at these visible clinical signs, but seeks out anything that seems strange, any unusual events, anything at all out of the ordinary in the description of this case. To do so, he seeks to uncover the connections between words on the basis of things that have been effaced or lost. He pursues the hidden, the masked, the details and clues, by the same method as in analysis...

His method was already that of psychoanalysis, which he was in the process of inventing, based on his belief in the existence of a psychological unconscious. Unlike Boissarie, he did not believe either in a supernatural power, in God or in the devil, and unlike Charcot, he did not relate this case to others. He did not standardize cases and smooth off their rough edges: on the contrary, he painstakingly dissected them in search of the dissimilar and the dissonant. First of all, he wonders why this pact with the devil is not made in return for either magic, pleasure or money! This seems to him illogical and absurd for a man who is staking his soul.[30] For the artist promises in the first pact in 1669 (signed in ink) to devote himself to this master for nine years as though he were his own son, while in the second, signed in blood in the same year, he likewise promises to be Satan's own son and to belong to him body and soul in nine years' time.[31] Freud also notes the changing representation of the devil, who becomes increasingly frightening: first he appears as a respectable bourgeois with a black dog at his side, then as a creature with horns, eagle's talons and bat's wings, and finally as a flying dragon. He notes the importance of the number nine (which he would long associate with femininity and moth-

25 Freud, 'A Seventeenth-Century Demonological Neurosis'.

26 Freud adds in a note that this confession may be related to the encouragement of the priest who had 'suggested' this explanation, but he does not dwell on this point. Freud, *Une névrose démoniaque*, 12.

27 He enjoyed good health from 15 January to 11 October 1678.

28 Freud, *Une névrose démoniaque*, 26-27. He returns in May 1678.

29 Ibid., 9.

30 Ibid., 13.

31 The meaning of this for Freud is that the painter, who has lost all desire and ability to work after his father's death, finds in the devil (who appears to him – on the first occasion at least – as a respectable bourgeois of a certain age) a substitute for his father.

erhood); finally and most importantly, he postulates that the steps which are described have a logic that must be deciphered. These symptoms presented in the manuscript as a sign of diabolical possession are for Freud the sign of a psychological disorder that he calls *demonological* neurosis ('neurosis' not being meant in the neurological sense). He claims that these phenomena, interpreted in the seventeenth century as related to the devil, must now be interpreted as neuroses related to psychological forces, wicked, condemned desires springing from rejected, repressed impulses. Evil no longer comes from outside but from within, from the depths of our own psyche.[32]

Freud introduces two radical interpretative innovations here. Firstly, he revisits the meaning of the simulation of illness, which was often alleged in the case of hysteria, with the suggestion that the patient had something to gain from the illness.[33] He takes up the Christian idea of the patient's responsibility during his or her illness, but excludes notions of morality and sin. Secondly, he shows that the causality of evil is not external but internal. As such, Freud's approach seems to me similar to that of Pasteur who, in the 1860s, replaced external, air-borne miasmata with microbes – a concept for which he had great difficulty in gaining acceptance from his fellow-scientists; the struggle faced by Pasteur and his supporters was far from over by the end of the nineteenth century. Man, therefore, could not only be destroyed by the incursions of creatures taking possession of his body but also, according to Freud, by the power of the effects of some hidden psychological element within, and this was even more disturbing. The psychoanalyst thus reintroduced an economy of emotions and revived in a new form the theory of passions, which for the early *aliénistes* Philippe Pinel and Étienne Esquirol were a major cause of insanity. In this respect he opposed Charcot, who with his breakdown of *hysteria major* into four periods thought he had resolved the question of the place of feelings and passions in hysteria by aligning the third phase, that of 'passionate attitudes', with the previous two thus preventing an emotion-based interpretation by focusing on the neurological.[34]

This revelation of the role of the emotions allowed Freud to argue that Haitzmann's feelings about his father were an ambivalent combination of tenderness, hostility and defiance, but also to deduce from them a history of the religious beliefs of mankind.[35] In the Freudian approach, the history of humans could be related to their psychological make-up, their beliefs and their imaginings, and the changes that had taken place in these could be under-

32 Freud, *Une névrose démoniaque*, 6.

33 Although he mentions the possibility that the painter is 'a simulator and a faker, and not possessed' as 'the boundaries between neurosis and simulation are known to be uncertain'. Freud, *Une névrose démoniaque*, 26. However, the journal written by Haitzmann is certainly a veracious depiction of neurosis.

34 Trillat, 'Introduction'.

35 Freud, *Une névrose démoniaque*, 16. Note by Freud: see *Totem and Taboo* and, for the details, Th. Reik, *Probleme der Religions psychologie* (Problems of Religious Psychology), 1, 1919.

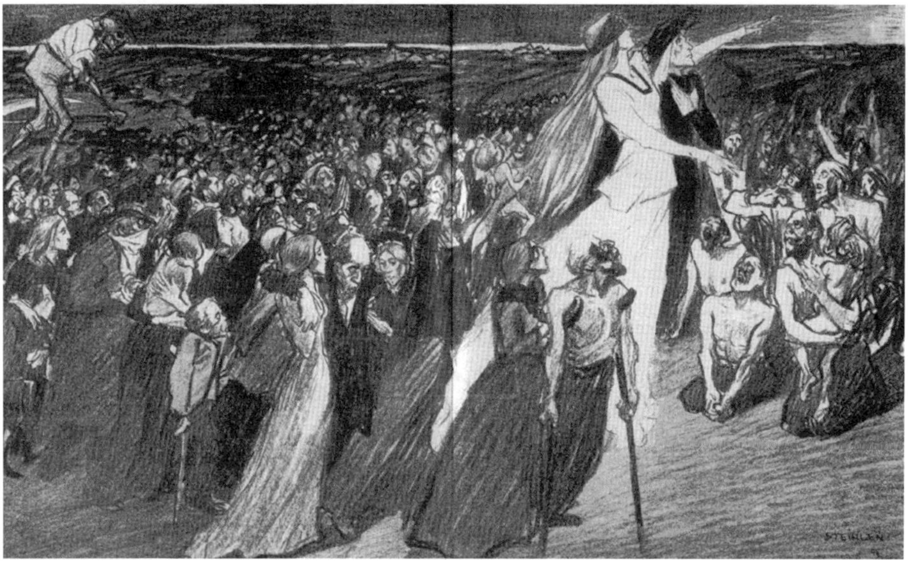

'Lourdes, allégorie de Steinlen'.
[Gil Blas, *22 April 1894*]

stood. Freud postulated that the passage of time would tend to fragment or conceal the traces of a primitive prototype, by a constant process of modification, exactly as also occurred for individuals (as he explained at greater length in *Totem and Taboo* in 1913). In this way, he undermined the foundations of religion, and especially of the monotheistic religions. In *Une névrose démoniaque*, he rewrote the history of religion, identifying a series of primitive foundations that men concealed and then forget about so that they could evolve and grow, just as individuals did.[36] Freud's disagreement with the Catholic doctors was absolute in this field. Belief had no place in analytic therapy, since it was merely a form of neurosis. Haitzmann's neurosis in the seventeenth century was clear, according to Freud, because it assumed a diabolical mask which seemed anachronistic in the early twentieth century. Thus, for Freud, the further back in time one went, the more evident neuroses became; just as the neuroses of childhood became buried in adulthood and could only be uncovered through in-depth investigation, so the neuroses of ages past revealed themselves clearly in certain aspects, such as the diabolical, whereas today they were disguised as organic diseases. And Freud pointed out that behind the manifestations of hysteria in the representations that art has transmitted to us, one could discover (*pace* Charcot) their neurotic content if one only took the trouble.[37]

36 Freud, *Une névrose démoniaque*, 16. Note by Freud on the opposing qualities of the divine: see Th. Reik, *Der eigene und der fremde Gott* (*The Strange God and One's Own God.*) (Imago, Ill, 1923), in the chapter entitled: 'God and Devil'.

37 Freud, *Une névrose démoniaque*, 5-6. See also de Certeau, 'Ce que Freud fait de l'histoire'.

Thus Freud not only made the idea seem abstruse that progress in medical science would banish religious beliefs: he characterized such beliefs as a clear sign of a pathological condition.

Boissarie, Charcot and Freud all observed the same types of pathological signs – convulsions, visions, seizures and paralyses – and were led by them to examine religious belief and the supernatural. Their medical knowledge and their training in positive, experimental medicine had taught them to disregard such phenomena as incompatible with the scientific knowledge of their day. Yet each in his own way took on this encounter. Boissarie reconciled religious belief and science easily, as he was convinced of the lack of any contradiction between them and could therefore have faith and believe in scientific progress without any problem. Regarding the cases he studied, he took the view that either the illness and its spectacular effects were real and the healing could be classified as miraculous, or that there was manipulation, simulation and immorality on the part of both patient and doctor, and that in order to find healing, each needed to return to the path of dignity and self-respect. Charcot was concerned only with his patients' body and nerves. A radical positivist in the medical field, the only belief he expressed was in scientific progress, which would soon reveal a neurological explanation for the cures at Lourdes and provide the physiological keys to these therapeutic miracles. Freud, for his part, took a huge sidestep and changed the focus of observation. Under these physical signs, he uncovered purely psychological symptoms. These bodily phenomena revealed to him neuroses that could not be understood in terms either of a brain injury or of manipulation or simulation, but in terms of something repressed and hidden within the self. What is more, the verbal expression of this malaise was not timeless: descriptions of it were couched in the beliefs of the age in which they were given. In the eighteenth century, people believed in the power of the devil and God, while in the late nineteenth and early twentieth century, people believed in the power of science; in either case, belief was, for Freud, a neurosis. Freud's convictions thus distinguished him from Charcot and Boissarie, yet their threefold contribution altered both the interpretation and the formal manifestations of these exceptional physical phenomena, which soon disappeared from the medical landscape. The physical symptoms of Charcot's *hysteria major* became increasingly rare after the death of its discoverer. Although hysterics continued to make their body their symptom, this use of the body as a mode of expression was now examined in its relations with the psychological, for, from the 1890s onwards, most patients were treated with various forms of psychotherapy, including psychoanalysis. The ability to put one's malaise into words had a modifying, calming effect on bodily behaviour, but even so, Freud failed to convince his peers of the validity of psychoanalysis, and religious belief remained an unchallenged value to many doctors, far removed from any form of neurosis.

PROPHECIES OF PILGRIMAGE

THE RISE AND FALL OF MARIE BERGADIEU, THE ECSTATIC OF FONTET

SOFIE LACHAPELLE

In 1901, the *Guide national et catholique du voyageur en France*, a Catholic travel guide highlighting the religious pilgrimages, monuments, spas, and natural curiosities of France, made a passing mention of the small town of Fontet near Bordeaux. It was there that, in 1873, a farmer's wife named Marie Bergadieu (1829-1904) had supposedly been miraculously cured following a Marian apparition. Over the years, one could read, the apparitions had continued to occur, but as the prophecies associated with them had never come to pass, all was soon forgotten.[1] By the time the *Guide national et catholique du voyageur en France* was published, Bergadieu was 72 years old. In a thousand-page book, her story had been told in a mere ten lines. But for a few years in the 1870s, the interest in Bergadieu had been significant, and she attracted many believers from her region and beyond. On 8 December 1873, the day of the Feast of the Immaculate Conception, for example, between one thousand and three thousand visitors had travelled to the farm to witness Bergadieu experience an apparition.[2] In the months following her miraculous recovery and the initial apparition, pamphlets encouraging pilgrims to visit Fontet were published; physicians came to examine and test the visionary; and while the Catholic Church itself kept its distance, many in the local clergy and beyond certainly showed enthusiasm for Bergadieu and her claims.

As time passed, Mary continued to appear in Fontet. From her initial laments about blasphemy and lack of prayer around the country, her messages

1 *Guide national et catholique du voyageur en France*, 850, 852.

2 See, for example, 'Chronique', *Le Temps*, 13 December 1873, 2 and Portets, *Lettres sur la voyante de Fontet. Première série*, 17.

turned political. Her prophecies as relayed by Bergadieu became precise: before the end of 1874; the Count of Chambord would rise to the French throne as Henri V. Frédéric de Bray (1817-1889), ex-Jesuit and founder of the Notre-Dame-des-Anges archiconfrery in Pourvouville, would become pope two years after the death of Pius IX (r. 1846-1878).[3] As for Fontet, a church would soon be built where the farm now stood, and within a few years, the town would become an important site of pilgrimage comparable to Lourdes. Over time, the phenomena continued to evolve. Seven months after her recovery, Bergadieu began to experience a state of trance in the minutes or hours preceding her conversations with the apparition. The following year, stigmata appeared, accompanied by pains of crucifixion. Later still, claims would be made that Bergadieu could on occasion materialize the communion wafer in her mouth and experience what was described as a state of mystical communion. From the spring of 1873 to early 1875, believers travelled to Fontet in great numbers. At times, processions were organized through Bergadieu's bedroom. Pilgrims slowly entered through one door and exited the other while Bergadieu kneeled in a state of ecstasy, immobile, her eyes completely open and her hands joined in prayer, sometimes left alone, other times poked and pinched by visiting physicians.[4]

In the 1870s, claims of Marian apparitions and other such phenomena, if extraordinary, were not entirely uncommon. Scholars have written on the growing occurrences of visions and prophecies in the second half of the nineteenth century, pointing to the numerous occasions in which visionaries, mostly poorer children and young women from the countryside, claimed to have seen and conversed with Mary (or, as they often referred to her, the Virgin Mary or the Blessed Virgin). In France, the apparitions and subsequent pilgrimages to La Salette (1846), Lourdes (1858), and Pontmain (1871) put corporeal experiences of faith at the forefront of consciousness for many believers. And it is not just Marian apparitions and prophecies, but also miracle-cures, episodes of ecstasies, pains of crucifixion, stigmata, and demonic possessions that scholars see occurring with more frequency during this period.[5] What did these visions, prophecies, and physical phenomena mean to those who experienced them, to their family, their community, their local priest, to the pilgrims who travelled to witness them, the physicians who came to test them,

3 On Notre-Dame-des Anges and de Bray, see Deville, *Notice historique sur la dévotion de Notre-Dame des Anges*.

4 For example, see Portets, *Lettres sur la voyante de Fontet. Deuxième série*, 59-61. On Bergadieu, see Maître, *Mystique et féminité*, 354-359.

5 For example, see Bouflet and Boutry, *Un signe dans le ciel*; Carroy, *Le mal de Morzine*; Corrado Pope, 'Immaculate and Powerful'; Devlin, *The Superstitious Mind*; Edelman, *Voyantes, guérisseuses et visionnaires*; Harris, 'Possession on the Borders'; Id., *Lourdes*; Kselman, *Miracles and Prophecies*; Lachapelle, 'Between Miracle and Sickness'; Maire, *Les possédés de Morzine*; Mayeur, 'Mgr Dupanloup et Louis Veuillot devant les "prophéties contemporaines" en 1874', and Zimdars-Swartz, *Encountering Mary*.

the critiques who vehemently attacked them, and all of those who read about them in newspapers, periodicals, and books of the time?

This chapter explores the public and collective experiences of Bergadieu's claims paying particular attention to the initial pilgrimage that rapidly developed in Fontet. It situates Bergadieu and her phenomena in the religious and political context of the early years of the French Third Republic and argues that, for a time, Fontet functioned as a site where religious and scientific performances, political and social anxieties, and grassroots devotion came together to create a sense of expectation and possibilities: royalist possibilities for a repentant France following a century of political unrest, commercial possibilities for a town that might just become a national site of pilgrimage, and spiritual possibilities for the pilgrims who travelled near and far to witness Bergadieu's phenomena. At the same time, Fontet could also be seen as a site of potential threat for a Church facing a growing number of visionaries and worried about the subversive potential some of their claims could hold. So while Bergadieu's fame was short-lived – by 1901, the *Guide national et catholique du voyageur en France* would present her story as no more than a passing curiosity – the initial enthusiasm and early pilgrimage that rapidly developed around her suggest the extent to which exceptional corporeal experiences of faith had permeated the French religious and political landscape of the period.

News of a miraculous recovery and a coming king

Telling the story of Marie Bergadieu is not an easy task. Accounts contradict themselves on some important facts, namely the exact nature of the disease that led to her miraculous recovery, whether or not she had experienced prior visions, and even whether she was the only one in her household to witness the apparitions. What sources do agree on is that Marie Bergadieu, also known as Berguille, was born in 1829 in the town of Loupiac, situated about 50 kilometres southeast of Bordeaux, that she came from a family of tenant farmers and that, at the age of twenty one, she married a tenant farmer (Bernard Josseaume, 1820-1891) and moved with him to Noaillac (40 kilometres southeast of Loupiac). In 1856, she and her family returned to Loupiac and finally settled in Fontet, a small commune close by. The Josseaumes had three children, Cathérine (1853), Pierre (1855) and Jean (1858). In 1871, Bergadieu lost her daughter, a tragic event that greatly affected her. At the onset of the apparitions, Bergadieu was said to live with her husband, her two

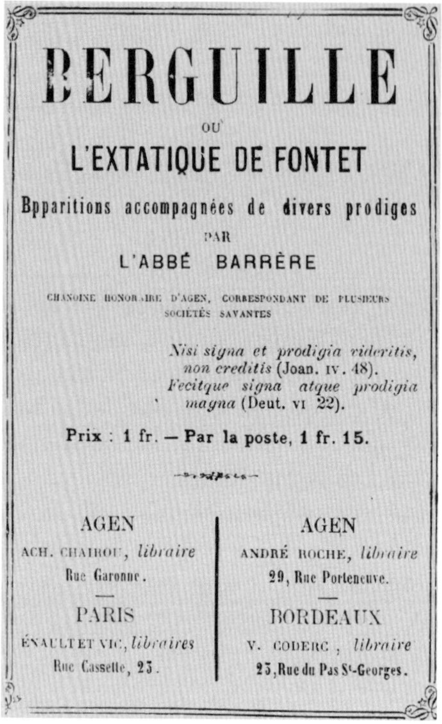

BERGUILLE

OU

L'EXTATIQUE DE FONTET

Apparitions accompagnées de divers prodiges

PAR

L'ABBÉ BARRÈRE

CHANOINE HONORAIRE D'AGEN, CORRESPONDANT DE PLUSIEURS SOCIÉTÉS SAVANTES

Nisi signa et prodigia videritis, non creditis (Joan. IV. 48).
Fecitque signa atque prodigia magna (Deut. VI 22).

Prix : 1 fr. — Par la poste, 1 fr. 15.

AGEN
ACH. CHAIROU, *libraire*
Rue Garonne.

PARIS
ÉNAULT ET VIC, *libraires*
Rue Cassette, 23.

AGEN
ANDRÉ ROCHE, *libraire*
29, Rue Porteneuve.

BORDEAUX
V. CODERC, *libraire*
23, Rue du Pas Sᵗ-Georges.

Title page of Joseph Barrère. Berguille, ou l'extatique de Fontet: Apparitions accompagnées de divers prodiges. Paris/Bordeaux, 1875.
[Paris, Bibliothèque nationale de France]

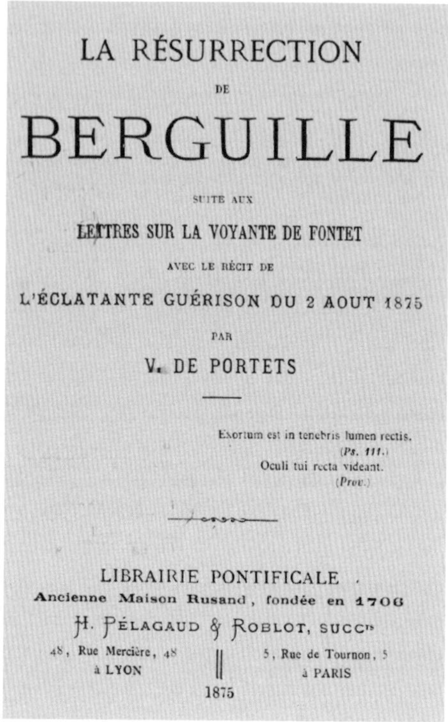

LA RÉSURRECTION

DE

BERGUILLE

SUITE AUX

LETTRES SUR LA VOYANTE DE FONTET

AVEC LE RÉCIT DE

L'ÉCLATANTE GUÉRISON DU 2 AOUT 1875

PAR

V. DE PORTETS

Exortum est in tenebris lumen rectis.
(*Ps. 111.*)
Oculi tui recta videant.
(*Prov.*)

LIBRAIRIE PONTIFICALE
Ancienne Maison Rusand, fondée en 1700
H. PÉLAGAUD & ROBLOT, SUCCᴿˢ
48, Rue Mercière, 48
à LYON
5, Rue de Tournon, 5
à PARIS
1875

Title page of V. de Portets. La résurrection de Berguille, suite aux Lettres sur la voyante de Fontet, avec le récit de l'éclatante guérison du 2 août 1875. Lyon/Paris, 1875.
[Paris, Bibliothèque nationale de France]

sons, her niece (nicknamed Tapiotte), and her niece's young daughter, Hermance.[6]

On her physical appearance, her intelligence, and her mental stability, accounts differ. A sympathetic account from 1874 described Bergadieu as tall and thin with beautiful, soft, and investigative eyes, calmness, and intelligence. Writing the same year, a medical student described her as taller than average, almost excessively thin, with a face older than her years, deep wrinkles, a hoarse voice, a sad smile, veiled eyes, all signs of prolonged illness and a morbid state.[7] Bergadieu was described by her supporters as either unable to read or reading very little but capable of expressing herself well. She spoke

6 See, for example, Ferrand, *La vérité touchant Berguille*, 12-13; Portets, *Lettres sur la voyante de Fontet. Première série*, 6; *La résurrection de la France et le châtiment de la Prusse*, 47, and Barrère, *Berguille, ou l'extatique de Fontet*, 8-9. Some of the biographical details are also taken from Maître, *Mystique et féminité*, 354.

7 Ferrand, *La vérité touchant Berguille*, 12 and Monydar, *Un doute sur la voyante de Fontet*, 4-5.

with 'simplicity, moderation and good sense; nothing in her suggests an exalted imagination or an impended intelligence; her air and her words indicate the greatest of sincerity', recalled one of her supporters.[8] In contrast to his wife, Josseaume was said to speak almost no French. He was also unable to read or write. Hermance, the daughter of Bergadieu's niece, also was said to speak mostly patois.[9]

Most accounts do not elaborate on Bergadieu's life before 1873 and her story tends to start in early that year when severe stomach pains forced her to stay in bed. Stomach cancer is generally mentioned as the cause of such pain (although there is some disagreement in the sources as to the nature and the severity of the illness).[10] What is generally agreed upon is that by April 1873 Bergadieu could no longer keep any food or drink and that her physician, Dr Béchade, felt he could do nothing further to help his patient. On 21 April, putting her faith in the hands of Mary, Bergadieu drank holy water from Lourdes and claimed to feel better right away. For the next eight days, she did not eat and continued to drink only the waters of Lourdes. Then, during the night of 27 April, Bergadieu reported seeing a light and a 'beautiful lady', bare foot and wearing a long white dress, her head covered with a white veil through which her long blonde hair was visible. The lady moved to the foot of the bed, came closer and put her hand on Bergadieu's mouth before disappearing. Not only was Bergadieu convinced that she had seen the Virgin Mary, she also thought that she would soon be cured. Still, her state seemed to worsen, she received the last sacraments that morning. The next night, the 'lady' returned. This time, the apparition confirmed that she was in fact the 'Immaculate Virgin'. Mary revealed that Bergadieu would indeed be cured after taking communion. Upon waking up the next morning, Bergadieu asked her priest for communion but was told that she was too sick for it. On the third night, Mary came back and lifted up parts of the sky to show Bergadieu that her deceased daughter was now in Heaven. The next morning, Bergadieu asked again and this time was allowed to take communion. Within fifteen minutes, she felt good enough to get out of bed and eat a little. And even though she had not eaten for days, as the story would often be retold, by noon she was back to work around the house.[11]

From then on, the visions continued to occur. By mid-August, Mary had already appeared twenty-seven times to Bergadieu. According to devotional

8 Portets, *Lettres sur la voyante de Fontet. Première série*, 6.

9 Ibid.

10 For example, the medical student Monydar doubted the validity of this diagnostic. He also brought attention to Bergadieu's fragile state of mind since the death of her daughter in 1871. See Monydar, *Un doute sur la voyante de Fontet*, 10-12.

11 This particular version can be found in Ferrand, *La vérité touchant Berguille*, 13-16. See also Portets, *Lettres sur la voyante de Fontet. Première série*, 6-8 for a similar account of the miracle-cure and the onset of the apparitions.

literature, these early apparitions could be short, sometimes lasting no more than two or three minutes, but at times lasting closer to an hour. Bergadieu could sense them coming. She would abandon her work, go back to her room and wait. Mary would appear; always dressed in white, her feet bare and her head covered by a white veil. She held a white rosary on her arm, which she asks Bergadieu to kiss each time. Although Bergadieu was initially the only one to see Mary, her niece's daughter, the young Hermance, claimed to have witnessed the fifteenth apparition. Mary had made a cross on her forehead, Hermance revealed. In subsequent apparitions, Hermance would claim that Mary had put her hand on her head or cheek. It was said that while Hermance did not confide easily about what she saw, when pushed, she provided the same description of the lady as her great-aunt.[12]

Not surprisingly, pilgrims rapidly began showing up in Fontet. Some would request that specific messages be conveyed to Mary, others wished to ask questions. At times, Mary would be presented with a rosary, a medal, or a scapular to bless. She was said to kindly answer and bless objects for believers, although she refused to consider secret messages provided to her in sealed envelopes.[13] During these early apparitions, Mary spoke against blasphemy and profanation and encouraged prayer and penance against the ills of the day. She revealed she had come to encourage conversions. Rapidly, she spoke of the future of Fontet. A church would be built here and become the centre of a great pilgrimage tradition. Fontet would become to the soul what Lourdes was to the body.[14] Later, the predictions would get more detailed: before the end of 1874, the bedroom would become a chapel. Within a few years, a basilica would be built nearby. It would become the most important pilgrimage site in the world.[15] But the messages were not just about Fontet. In May, they turned political. On 14 May, Mary announced that there would soon be a new government in France and after that the time would be for a Christian king to come to the throne once again. When the royalist (and Legitimist) Patrice de Mac-Mahon, Duke of Magenta (1808-1893), was announced as the President of the Republic ten days later, believers interpreted this as the change that had been predicted. Then, on 26 July, St Anne's Feast Day, Mary revealed that the future king of France would soon come and that he would be Henri V, the Count of Chambord, Legitimist pretender to the French throne. On 11 September 1873, Mary added that Henri V would come from the hand of God and not the will of men.[16]

12 Portets, *Lettres sur la voyante de Fontet. Première série*, 9-10 and Ferrand, *La vérité touchant Berguille*, 20.

13 Ibid., 11.

14 Ibid., 13.

15 Clauchai-Larsenal, *Berguille et Louise Lateau*, 28-29.

16 Portets, *Lettres sur la voyante de Fontet. Première série*, 13-14.

The possibility of a return to a monarchical system marked the early years of the Third Republic. Created following the collapse of the Second Empire, the Third Republic saw France through the crushing defeat in the Franco-Prussian War, the loss of Alsace-Lorraine, and the rise of the Paris Commune. Many saw it as a temporary government that would soon be replaced by a monarchy. But with royalists divided between the Legitimists (who supported the Bourbon pretender – the Count of Chambord), and the Orleanists (who supported the claimant of the Orléans branch of the royal family – the Count of Paris), a conservative republic managed to stay in place. Among the population, however, support for a royal France remained strong. In the countryside, visionaries like Bergadieu brought forth messages from Mary that France had not been abandoned but now needed to repent. After a century of revolutions, republicanism, revolts, and barricades, grassroots devotional movements expressed anxieties toward the modern world. In his work on nineteenth-century miracles and prophecies, Thomas Kselman points to a sense of guilt among the Catholics and a widespread belief that France was being punished for the sins of the Revolution. Following the defeat in the Franco-Prussian war and the violence associated with the Paris Commune, such anxieties ran rampant.[17] In January 1871, while the Prussian army was still advancing into France, a few village children from Pontmain saw the Virgin Mary in the sky one night. News of the apparition brought hope to many that France was not lost. The following year, children from the village of Neubois in Alsace (now part of the German Empire) claimed to have had a vision of Mary holding a sword and hitting the bowed heads of Prussian soldiers with force.[18] And, in 1873, the Breton Marie Julie Jahenny (1850-1941) revealed visions of the rise of the Great Catholic Monarch and the end of the world. Punishment would fall of France first, and then the rest of the world, she predicted. The times were indeed dark.

In Fontet, Mary made no secret of her displeasure with the times. On 10 October 1873, in front of fourteen witnesses, Bergadieu revealed she had been told that Mary would answer no requests that day. Instead, she asked people to pray. 'Tell everyone to pray a lot', she said. 'Pray for the salvation of France; because I will save it.' Mary deplored blasphemy and those who hoped to destroy everything in the world. Evil believed it had already won but 'Henri V will come and save France'.[19] Soon, a timeline was provided: 'We face a great political crisis, a supreme crisis; the more we pray the shorter it will be. Without fixing an exact month or day, I cannot, I affirm that Henri V will come back and rise on the throne of France in 1874. His accession will be

17 Kselman, *Miracles and Prophecies*, esp. 113-123.
18 On the Neubois apparitions and miracle-cures see Klein, 'The Virgin with the Sword'.
19 Portets, *Lettres sur la voyante de Fontet. Première série*, 15.

preceded and followed by great trouble that some great cities and mostly Paris will suffer.'[20]

For Legitimists, these apparitions and the royalist prophecies that often accompanied them were a topic of great interest. The journalist Adrien Péladan (1815-1890) wrote a number of works on these royalist prophecies and heavily promoted countryside visionaries, particularly Bergadieu and Jahenny who were said to be 'sisters in suffering'. (Later, when Bergadieu would begin to experience pains of crucifixion on Fridays, the two visionaries would claim to be able to see and communicate with each other throughout their ordeal).[21] *Le rosier de Marie*, a weekly journal featuring extraordinary religious phenomena, promoted Berguille and her legitimist prophecies. The journal also promoted the candidacy of Frédéric de Bray to the papacy.[22] Among the clergy, there were some who supported apparitions and prophecies including the abbé Jean-Marie Curicque of Metz who published *Voix prophétiques ou signes, apparitions et prédictions modernes* looking for signs of the end of times. The fact that *Voix prophétiques* went through five editions between 1870 and 1872 is evocative of the appeal that such literature held. While certainly not a sanctioned position within the Church – in fact, in 1872, Pius IX had indicated a certain reservation regarding the proliferation of modern prophecies – Curicque's position was nonetheless indicative of a strong current present in French Catholicism at the time.[23]

20 *La résurrection de la France et le châtiment de la Prusse*, 66. In the early 1870s, memories of the defeat in the Franco-Prussian war and the popular revolt of the Commune in Paris were still fresh, and Paris was seen by many Catholics as morally culpable. See, for example, Jonas, *France and the Cult of the Sacred Heart*, particularly chapters 6 and 7. According to Adrien Péladan, Bergadieu talked on many occasions of Paris as a damned city that would suffer. See, for example, Péladan, *(Suite à Dernier mot des Prophéties)*, 26-28.

21 Portets, *La résurrection de Berguille*, 29. See also Péladan, *Ma retraite du châtiment* and Id., *(Suite à Dernier mot des Prophéties)*. On Péladan, see Drouin, 'Un légitimiste mystique du XIXème siècle'.

22 Maître, *Mystique et féminité*, 355-357.

23 Curicque, *Voix prophétiques ou signes*. On Pius IX's declarations regarding modern prophecies, see Chabauty, *Les prophéties modernes vengées*, 27-33. On Curicque, see Multon, 'Faire de la politique du miracle'. On the various currents and nuances present in Catholicism in the second half of the nineteenth century, see Mayeur, 'Mgr Dupanloup et Louis Veuillot'; Multon, 'Catholicisme intransigeant et culture prophétique' and Id., 'Prophétesses et prophécies'.

Pilgrims and physicians travel to Fontet

From the spring to the fall of 1873, Bergadieu continued to receive and relay the political and spiritual messages of Mary. During these apparitions, Bergadieu was described by witnesses as absorbed, moving her lips and standing still as if talking and listening to someone.[24] In November, a change occurred. On the 21st of the month, she experienced her first state of ecstasy. As she kneeled and joined her hands, she entered a trance. When burned on a finger with a candle or poked with needles on her face and hands to the point of bleeding, she remained immobile and serene, as witnessed by a crowd of one hundred and thirty-four observers.[25] On 25 November, Mary informed Bergadieu that further experiments could be planned for 8 December, the day of the Feast of the Immaculate Conception, as she would appear at some point between noon and one in the afternoon. According to Bergadieu, Mary had revealed that 'Many doubters will come to this apparition. They must be allowed to approach; those that are convinced do not need to be so close. There will be a lot of priests; a lot of physicians will come as well: it is necessary that it is so.'[26]

By all account, a large crowd came to witness the apparition of 8 December. The newspaper *Le Temps* estimated one thousand were present, remarking on 'public credulity' and hallucinations that would likely make Bergadieu feel at home at the Saint-Anne or de la Salpêtrière hospitals.[27] Writing under the pseudonym V. de Portets, Victor Lac de Bosredon more generously estimated a crowd of three thousand to have travelled to Fontet to stand outside the farm while, in her bedroom, Bergadieu fell to her knees and entered a state of ecstasy. In front of witnesses, Mary appeared to Bergadieu and again warned believers of dangers and an 'eminent crisis'. She emphasized the need for prayer. Henri V would come soon, she told Bergadieu to reassure everyone again as she blessed them. As asked, physicians were present and ready to test Bergadieu. Dr Bonnefroy of Langon and Dr Béchade of Puybarban (who knew Bergadieu since 1871 and had published a letter in *La Gironde* two months earlier stating that he believed Bergadieu to be a *monomane*) were both in the room and testified that Bergadieu was indeed in a trance in which she had become insensitive to external stimulus including pain.[28] In the coming months, physicians would continue to observe and test Bergadieu. On 24 December, for example, Dr Béchade returned to Fontet, this time accompanied by Dr Bensse

24 Portets, *Lettres sur la voyante de Fontet. Première série*, 12.
25 Ibid., 16-17 and *La résurrection de la France et le châtiment de la Prusse*, 55-56.
26 Portets, *Lettres sur la voyante de Fontet. Première série*, 17.
27 'Chronique', *Le Temps*, 13 December 1873, 2.
28 Portets, *Lettres sur la voyante de Fontet. Première série*, 17-19, 23-24 and *La résurrection de la France et le châtiment de la Prusse*, 59. Dr Béchade's letter of 12 October 1873 to *La Gironde* was published in Clauchai-Larsenal, *Berguille et Louise Lateau*, 35. See also Maître, *Mystique et féminité*, 358.

of Bordeaux. Both declared the ecstasy to be real and Bergadieu to appear healthy and sane.[29]

By the 1870s, it had become clear that Marian apparitions could have tremendous economic, social, and spiritual consequences for a town and a region. In Lourdes, the apparitions of 1858 had led to a major pilgrimage tradition. Within ten years, a train station had been built while newly opened shops sold souvenirs, postal cards, and mini dioramas. By the early 1870s, this once poor and isolated community had become a site where faith, tourism, and consumerism intertwined.[30] In Fontet, Mary continued to assure pilgrims and town inhabitants alike that a pilgrimage would develop on the site. 'Here will be my sanctuary', she was reported to have said again on 18 January 1874 in the *Journal des débats politiques et littéraires*.[31] There is some evidence that the potential economic importance of Bergadieu's experiences was apparent at least to some in her community. Reporting on his visit to Fontet in 1874, journalist Albert Moisnard mentioned that the grocers had now begun selling medals and rosaries, that a merchant of religious objects had come to town and set up an altar in Bergadieu's bedroom, and that a woman from Fontet had initially helped spread word of Bergadieu's apparitions by recording the revelations into notebooks which she then circulated beyond Fontet.[32] That some in Fontet encouraged and even helped Bergadieu seems possible. Relating their own visit to Fontet in 1875, Bordeaux physicians Emile Mauriac and Henri Verdalle recalled that upon arriving at the La Réole train station late they had been reassured by a pious woman present not to worry as Bergadieu usually could predict the arrival of visitors and thus wait for them before she began. While surprised, the two physicians then overheard a conversation that led them to believe that Bergadieu had likely been informed of their visit by the postman's daughter.[33]

Of course, a pilgrimage site would need reports of miracles. In Lourdes, the grotto was filled with abandoned crushes, an impressive visual testimony to the promises of the sanctuary. In Fontet, pilgrims also rapidly began to talk of miracles. Already in December 1873, a man said to be possessed by a demon had been present in Bergadieu's room during one of the apparitions. While not cured, his state was said to have improved following his visit.[34] Then, on Christmas Eve of the same year, a neighbour described as sceptical reported having seen a white light illuminating the farm while Bergadieu was expe-

29 Portets, *Lettres sur la voyante de Fontet. Première série*, 28.
30 Kaufman, *Consuming Visions*, 2-3. On Lourdes, see also Harris, *Lourdes*.
31 *Journal des débats politiques et littéraires*, 17 February 1874, 2.
32 Moisnard, 'Berguille. La voyante de Fontet', 2.
33 Mauriac and Verdalle, *Étude médicale sur l'extatique de Fontet*, 39.
34 Mary had also declared that he would soon be cured: Portets, *Lettres sur la voyante de Fontet. Première série*, 30-31).

riencing a vision of the Holy Family inside.[35] Claims of white light or flames dancing in the night sky continued to be heard in the following years.[36] At the same time, some visitors claimed to have been cured from various conditions including a blind man who had already travelled to Lorette, Verdelais, and Lourdes without success but was said to have regained his sight during his stay in Fontet.[37]

Starting in 1874, pilgrims wishing to visit Fontet could rely on *La vérité touchant Berguille* by Camille Ferrand to organize their trip. Ferrand described his own visit to Fontet and included touristic information. Starting with the sixty kilometre train ride from Bordeaux to La Réole (like Lourdes before Bernadette, Fontet did not have its own train station), Ferrand informed his readers of the sites worthy of their attention: the former castle of Saint Paulin here, a spot visited by Catherine of Medici or Jeanne d'Albret there. In Villenave-d'Ornon, one of the best white wines of the Gironde was cultivated; in Caudaujac was a church with curious roman capitals; Saint-Médard-d'Eyrans was the birth place of Montesquieu, and so on. Arriving in La Réole, pilgrims were encouraged to visit some of the sites: the beautiful Gothic church, the Benedictine monastery, the Couvent des Cordeliers, the Château des Quatre-Sœurs, and a number of preserved medieval buildings. From there, a short three-kilometre walk would bring them to Bergadieu's home, a modest farm on a hill.[38]

Once at the farm, visitors would hope to witness Bergadieu in the midst of one of her trances. Describing the 2 February 1874 apparition in front of more than two thousand pilgrims, one awestruck observer wrote:

> I will not attempt to describe the beauty of the expression of Berguille's face: it would be impossible. At times an unexplainable smile illuminated her traits: her lips would stir as if she had pronounced a prayer or professed some answer, then she would lower her head; other times a profound sadness would come over her face and her eyes would fill themselves with tears but, extraordinarily, these tears, far from running along her cheeks, disappeared under her eyelids as if by enchantment... . I will not enter into details on all of trials to which physicians subjected the body of the poor Sightseer, trials that in no way changed her attitude. No matter how they pinched her, pinned her, pulled her

35 Barrère, *Berguille, ou l'extatique de Fontet*, 104-105.

36 Ibid., 105-107.

37 Barrère reproduces a number of letters from visitors: Barrère, *Berguille, ou l'extatique de Fontet*, 70-88.

38 Ferrand, *La vérité touchant Berguille*, 7-11, 25 and Daurelle, *Les évènements de Fontet d'après les principes de St Thomas*, vii.

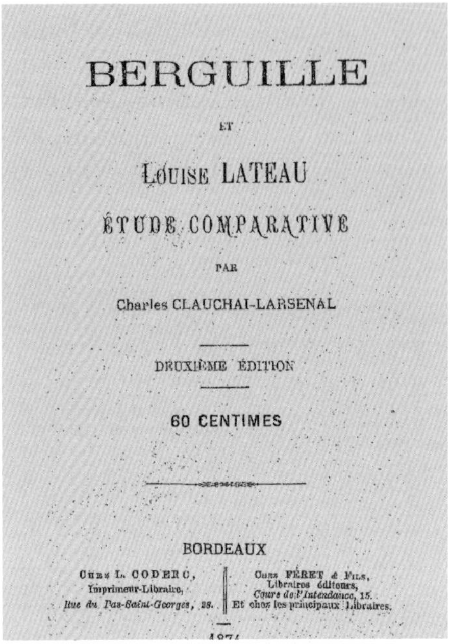
BERGUILLE

ET

LOUISE LATEAU

ÉTUDE COMPARATIVE

PAR

Charles CLAUCHAI-LARSENAL

DEUXIÈME ÉDITION

60 CENTIMES

BORDEAUX

CHEZ L. CODERC, Imprimeur-Libraire, *Rue du Pas-Saint-Georges*, 28.	CHEZ FÉRET & FILS, Libraires éditeurs, *Cours de l'Intendance*, 15. Et chez les principaux Libraires.

1874

Title page of Charles Clauchai-Larsenal. Berguille et Louise Lateau. Étude comparative. *Bordeaux, 1874.* [*Leuven, Maurits Sabbebibliotheek*]

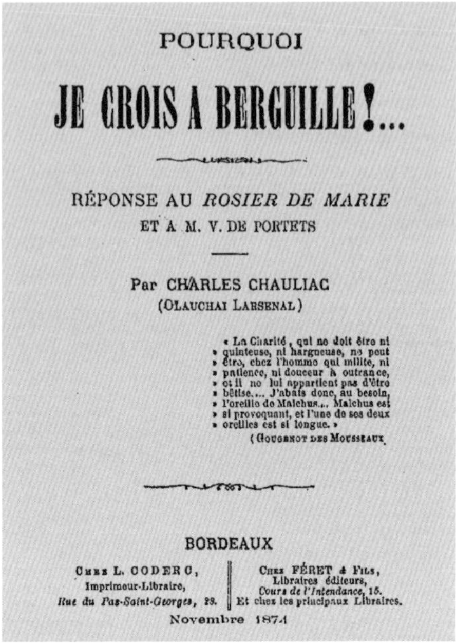
POURQUOI

JE CROIS A BERGUILLE !...

RÉPONSE AU *ROSIER DE MARIE*

ET A M. V. DE PORTETS

Par CHARLES CHAULIAC

(CLAUCHAI LARSENAL)

« La Charité, qui ne doit être ni
» quinteuse, ni hargneuse, ne peut
» être, chez l'homme qui milite, ni
» patience, ni douceur à outrance,
» et il ne lui appartient pas d'être
» bêtise.... J'abats donc, au besoin,
» l'oreille de Malchus.... Malchus est
» si provoquant, et l'une de ses deux
» oreilles est si longue. »
(GOUGENOT DES MOUSSEAUX.

BORDEAUX

CHEZ L. CODERC, Imprimeur-Libraire, *Rue du Pas-Saint-Georges*, 28.	CHEZ FÉRET & FILS, Libraires éditeurs, *Cours de l'Intendance*, 15. Et chez les principaux Libraires.

Novembre 1874

Title page of Charles Clauchai-Larsenal. Pourquoi je crois à Berguille! Réponse au Rosier de Marie et à M.V. de Portets. *Bordeaux, 1874* [*Leuven, Maurits Sabbebibliotheek*]

> hair, pinched her nose to prevent her from breathing, she remained insensitive.[39]

Reporting on his visit the same day, another impressed observer recalled five or six physicians present and testing Bergadieu's insensitivity by pulling her hair, burning a match close to her right eye, putting fire under her finger, violently throwing water on her face, and digging hair pins into her shoulders.[40] To confirm that the apparitions were not the work of the devil, holy water was also said to have been thrown on Bergadieu to no effect.[41]

In the spring of 1874, Bergadieu began to experience pains of crucifixion. From then on, she would receive the pain on most Fridays, following the Stations of the Cross to the crucifixion, her body rigid with small stigmata. Reports from observers suggest very minor stigmata. Portets talked of cavities on each hand (with the left one more pronounced) and a double cavity on the

39 Observation of J. Edouard Geneste as reported by Portets in *Lettres sur la voyante de Fontet. Deuxième série*, 29-30.

40 *La résurrection de la France et le châtiment de la Prusse*, 62-64.

41 Portets, *Lettres sur la voyante de Fontet. Deuxième série*, 64.

left foot.[42] The Catholic sympathizer and wine merchant in Bordeaux Charles Chauliac (writing under the pseudonym Charles Clauchai-Larsenal) travelled to Fontet in June 1874 to witness the stigmata and saw no blood on the hands, feet, or forehead. On the palms, he witnessed nothing more than a little pinkish sweat.[43] The feet, however, exhibited more. On the top of each foot were purplish forms three centimetres in length by one and a half centimetres in width. At the centre of the bruise of the left foot, a small scratch could be seen. No blood was visible but a few drops of water appeared to emanate from the scratch.[44] During the same visit, Chauliac also tested the state of insensitivity. Along with Dr Béchade, who was again present, he pinched Bergadieu's arm enough to draw blood and observed no reaction. It was as if she had not noticed even if, an hour later, a mark remained visible.[45]

In 1874, Chauliac wrote an entire book comparing Bergadieu to Louise Lateau (1850-1883), one of the most famous stigmatic of the second half of the nineteenth century. In 1868, Lateau had begun to experience trances and stigmata in her village of Bois d'Haine in Belgium. Since then, and until her death in 1883, she continued to experience her phenomena every Friday (and sometimes on religious holidays). Over the years, Lateau had attracted countless pilgrims, Church officials, and physicians to her house. She had been the subject of medical commission, observed by members of the Académie royale de médecine de Belgique, and had been the topic of one of Dr Antoine Imbert-Gouyebeyre's two volumes on stigmatization (published in 1873 as Bergadieu's apparitions were just beginning). Having visited both Bois d'Haine and Fontet, Chauliac commented on the similarities between both women and attested to their good faith, simple and naïve piety, and disinterest with money. But while Lateau did not appear to enjoy her fame and refused to make prophecies, Bergadieu publically announced her phenomena and told of her visions and her experiences to anyone who wished to hear in great details.[46]

Bergadieu's prophecies turned out to be her greatest weakness. The initial interest in her claims, the willingness of physicians to declare her trances genuine, the enthusiasm of her supporters, and the cautious silence of the Church on her case, all of this helped to further her initial popularity and the belief in the validity of her phenomena. As the months went by and prophecies about the Count of Chambord and Frédéric de Bray continued, however,

42 Id., *La résurrection de Berguille*, 27.

43 Clauchai-Larsenal, *Berguille et Louise Lateau*, 15, 19. See also Clauchai-Larsenal, *Pourquoi je crois à Berguille*. On Chauliac's profession, see Maître, *Mystique et féminité*, 358.

44 Clauchai-Larsenal, *Berguille et Louise Lateau*, 20.

45 Ibid., 22.

46 Ibid., 32-33. Lateau was asked, at least once, to make a prediction of the Count of Chambord but refused to answer. On Louise Lateau, see Lachapelle, 'Between Miracle and Sickness'.

doubts began to creep in, even among supporters.[47] By December 1874, anxious travellers were still arriving in Fontet, but some were beginning to suspect the devil of causing the apparitions. On 22 December, Mary appeared to Bergadieu with a black crucifix on her chest and told the visionary that the time had come for her to reveal a secret to President Mac-Mahon. On 27 December, Bergadieu travelled to Paris where she unsuccessfully tried to get an audience with the French President before the end of the year. She came back to Fontet on 1 January, having entrusted a letter for the President to a royalist supporter.[48] But it was now 1875 and the Republic was still in place. Many were disappointed.

While the apparitions and the trances continued into 1875, the enthusiasm for Bergadieu had thawed. Back in December, Cardinal Ferdinand Donnet, archbishop of Bordeaux, had answered a query from the publisher of the Librairie Pontificale in Lyon on whether or not to publish a pamphlet on Bergadieu (presumably Portets's *La résurrection de Berguille*, published in 1875). The events occurring in Fontet, he had written, had been examined with seriousness and impartiality and did not warrant further consideration.[49] Wanting to end the 'pilgrimage to Fontet' as it had begun to be described over in Bordeaux, the archbishop decided that no visit to Bergadieu's farm could occur without special permission.[50] But the matter was not closed for all, even among the clergy. In *Berguille, ou l'extatique de Fontet* (1875), for example, l'abbé Joseph Barrère wrote of his reaction to the unrealized prophecy. Yes, he had been momentarily discouraged in January 1875, but the visions had continued. For him, this was an indication that the apparitions were not the work of the devil, who would have abandoned Bergadieu once the confusion had been established.[51] But why did Bergadieu claim that Henri V would rise to the throne by the end of 1874? In October 1875, Barrère was granted permission to travel to Fontet and seek an answer to his question. When asked, Bergadieu explained that Mary had told her that she had misinterpreted her words; she was uneducated and had failed to report the exact messages that had been revealed to her. Henri would rise but Mary had never been as clear as Bergadieu thought on when this would happen.[52]

47 On prophecies about Frédéric de Bray, see, for example, Clauchai-Larsenal, *Berguille et Louise Lateau*, 24-25.
48 Portets, *La résurrection de Berguille*, 12-14.
49 The letter is reproduced in 'La voyante de Fontet', *Annales catholiques*, 22 January 1875, 217-218.
50 Portets, *La résurrection de Berguille*, 14 and 'La destruction de Paris', *L'Echo du merveilleux*, 1 June 1905, 202.
51 Barrère, *Berguille, ou l'extatique de Fontet*, 6.
52 Ibid., 15-17.

Failed prophecies and forgotten pilgrimage

By 1875, Fontet had become significantly calmer. Gone were the long processions of pilgrims passing through the bedroom. For physicians, this made the task of testing Bergadieu easier. In June, a medical commission was unofficially put together by the vicar-general in Bordeaux. Drs Segay, Bulard, and Labarthe from Bordeaux, Dr Duprada from La Réole and Dr de Lentillac from Hure met in Fontet on Wednesday, 2 June and found Bergadieu in a state of ecstasy lasting since the previous Friday. Testing her insensitivity, they made Bergadieu smell ammonia, severely scratched her hands and arms, and rapidly moved a lancet towards her eye as if intending to pierce it. In vain, Bergadieu did not react. Nothing was able to break her trance except for a simple command in the name of the Holy Church, according to one witness present. While the results of the commission were said to have been favourable, a report was not produced.[53]

A little over a week later, the two editors of the *Gazette médicale de Bordeaux*, the physicians Mauriac and Verdalle, were also able to see Bergadieu. In *Étude médicale sur l'extatique de Fontet*, they related their visit to Fontet on 11 June and relayed some of the information they had obtained from Dr Béchade and others.[54] In their account of Bergadieu's life prior to 1873, Mauriac and Verdalle somewhat differed from others. For example, they mentioned one son rather than two, and discussed earlier demonic apparitions in Aillas (10 kilometres from Fontet), where Bergadieu supposedly lived from 1859 to 1865 (although this was not mentioned by any other author with the exception of the ones who likely took their biographical information directly from them). Mauriac and Verdalle claimed to have reliable witnesses who confirmed that, at the time she was living in Aillas, Bergadieu believed she was seeing the devil and often could be spotted outside at night pursuing him through the woods with a pitch fork. Later, after her daughter's death in 1871, she was said to have confided in Drs de Lentillac and Béchade separately that she was visited by her dead child every night.[55] As for her initial miraculous recovery, Mauriac and Verdalle explained that Dr Béchade had initially been called to Bergadieu's bed sight for violent stomach pains. While never witnessing her in the act of vomiting, he did confirm that he had been told by the patient and her family that she could not keep anything down. No matter what treatment he tried, Bergadieu still complained of vomiting everything. Dr Béchade recalled having asked the family for a sample of the vomit, telling

53 Barrère, who had been present for the work of the commission and its subsequent discussions, speculated that this was because two of the members, Segay and Labarthe believed the phenomena to be supernatural: Barrère, *Berguille, ou l'extatique de Fontet*, 53-61.

54 Mauriac and Verdalle, *Étude médicale sur l'extatique de Fontet*, 23.

55 Ibid., 11-13.

them that if it was black, it could indicate cancer of the stomach. From this comment to the family, the authors speculated, had come the tale of a miraculous recovery from a cancer of the stomach.[56]

Mauriac and Verdalle's own visit to Fontet took place with around fifteen witnesses present, mostly family members and neighbours. The two physicians arrived at the farm to find Bergadieu in bed claiming that her entire body had been in pain since the previous night. They were able to witness a state of ecstasy first hand, from the Stations of the Cross, to crucifixion, and finally the apparition of Mary. They monitored Bergadieu's pulse and tested her sensitivity with pinches, needles and electric shock. They tried to get her to smell ammonia and reported that she appeared to be holding her breath. They monitored her eye movements and pupil contractions. When sneaking up on her in an attempt to startle her, they observed that she moved a little despite claims of insensitivity. Moreover, the two physicians reported that Bergadieu had appeared to retain a sense of decency throughout the ecstasy, at times fixing her dress and her bed sheets. As well, no stigmata were noticed that day, although Dr Bulard from the medical commission earlier that month did confirm to them that he had seen something during his visit to Fontet.[57]

To explain their observations, Mauriac and Verdalle appealed to the previous claims of hysteria and pathological hallucinations: Bergadieu had seen the devil at a time when she was hearing stories about him in her little town. Then, once in a larger city, she saw her dead daughter. Now, more religious than ever and hearing all the stories from Lourdes, she saw Mary. After all, the newspapers were filled with talks of prophecies and imminent crisis. In this context, Bergadieu's visions were not particularly extraordinary. Besides, at their onset, the apparitions had occurred after a period of abstinence. Although she very likely did not suffer from stomach cancer, Bergadieu had been sick and weak for a while. She had also not eaten for eight days. Referring to studies on the stigmatic Louise Lateau, the two physicians suggested that abstinence had been key in provoking the visions (or hallucinations).[58] For them, Bergadieu suffered from an 'extraordinary neurosis' or a 'stigmatic neuropathy' most likely caused by '... a lesion of the bulb, congestion of the vaso-motor centre and respiratory centre, brought upon by an initial congestion of the optical layers'.[59] Science, the two physicians concluded, could go no further at this point.

While they made no accusation of fraud, Mauriac and Verdalle did conclude that at least some simulation had likely been involved in bringing about episodes of ecstasy and this for four reasons: 1) Bergadieu could predict the

56 Mauriac and Verdalle, *Étude médicale sur l'extatique de Fontet*, 13-14.
57 Ibid., 23-30, 56-57.
58 Ibid., 21, 33-37.
59 Ibid., 68.

onset of her trances with exactness; 2) at times, she had showed a sense of decency during her trances; 3) she appeared to be helped by others, whether consciously or not[60]; and 4) she used certain mechanisms to help induce her state of ecstasy – namely breathing techniques, concentration, and prayer. But while a crisis could be encouraged by these methods, both physicians believed while in a state of ecstasy, there had been no simulation.[61] The suggestion that parts of Bergadieu's experience were simulated was criticized by physician Claude Etienne Bourdin who published an unfavourable commentary on Mauriac and Verdalle's work in the *Annales médico-psychologiques*. Without meeting Bergadieu, he argued that her attacks were likely pathological and not at all under her control. Science, however, was not advanced enough to explain the phenomena further.[62] In *Études cliniques sur l'hystero-epilepsie ou grade hystérie*, the physician and professor of comparative anatomy Paul Richer agreed with Bourdin that there was no simulation involved; rather it was more likely a case of hystero-epilepsie, not unlike the ones that could be seen in the hospitals of the capital.[63]

By 1875, Bergadieu no longer made as many revelations. As for her previous incorrect ones, the humiliation she now endured because of them was a trial she said she was willing to bear. Her pains of crucifixion, ecstasies, and conversations with Mary continued and, in July 1875, began to be accompanied by a new phenomenon: the apparent materialization of the wafer in her mouth, a phenomenon also witnessed by supporters of Marie-Julie Jahenny.[64] Reporting on the apparition of 9 July 1875, Portets mentioned that a 'mystical communion' had been observed by fourteen witnesses.[65] Again on 16 July, an observer described a wafer of brilliant whiteness the size of a coin. During a trance, Bergadieu had first stuck her tongue out as if to show it was empty and then stuck it out a second time as if to show the wafer: '[t]he illusion was not possible. Berguille has received the holy communion, as always with the greatest respect and the most profound reverence', the observer recalled.[66]

By then, Bergadieu no longer attracted much attention outside her circle of staunch supporters and some in the medical community. If the early years

60 Ibid., 39. Mauriac and Verdalle believed that their visit had been announced to Bergadieu by the postman's daughter, thus encouraging the seer to wait for their arrival before starting.

61 Ibid., 38-47.

62 Bourdin, *L'extatique de Fontet*.

63 Richer, *Études cliniques sur l'hystero-epilepsie ou grade hystérie*, 319-320. On nineteenth-century French physicians and corporeal experiences of faith more broadly, see Harris, 'The "Unconscious" and Catholicism in France' and Szarbo, 'Seeing is Believing?' On French physicians of the period and Catholicism more generally, see Paul, *From Knowledge to Power*, 221-250.

64 Péladan, *Dernier mot des prophéties*, 160.

65 Portets, *La résurrection de Berguille*, 107.

66 Ibid., 111-112.

of the Third Republic had been marked by a desire of many for a return to a monarchical system, by the middle of the 1870s, it had become clear that a republic could work, even for royalists. As such, talks of monarchy became less frequent. In Fontet, both the prophecies of the rise of Henri V and of a basilica now looked unlikely. Time had shown Bergadieu's claims to be untrue. Ecclesiastics were forbidden to enter the Bergadieu farm. As for believers, they were strongly encouraged to abstain from the visit: 'If there are still some who, disregarding religious authority, rush to witness ridiculous, grotesques, or scandalous phenomena, it will now only concern those in charge of public order', one could read in the *Bulletin du diocèse de Reims* in 1876.[67]

In the following years, the apparitions and the prophecies continued. The crisis was eminent, a disaster would come: 'Poor France!... Poor Church!', Bergadieu lamented in September 1876.[68] As for Fontet, it seems Mary was still promising that it would become a centre of pilgrimage and prayer. 'This basilica will be the most beautiful in the universe!', Bergadieu revealed in August 1877.[69] While most had given up, a few still hoped, even within the Church. In 1878, the abbé Daurelle of Mende wrote of his travels to Fontet and his support for Bergadieu but was soon disciplined by the Church.[70] As for Royalist Adrien Péladan, he continued to publically support Bergadieu and reedited texts about the events taking place in Fontet at least as late as 1881.[71] In August 1883, however, even the staunchest of Legitimists had to accept the death of the Count of Chambord.

In his work on the German apparitions of 1876 in Marpingen, historian David Blackbourn outlined the typical phases for claims of Marian apparitions: first, a local event impacted the visionary or visionaries, their family members, their community, and their parish priest. In a second phase, pilgrims and curious began to show up bringing along the promise of a commercial exploitation. It is at this point that the political significance of the apparitions and the real or assumed social threats to public order would attract the attention of both civil and religious authorities. For Blackbourn, the vast majority of cases would collapse in this phase, either because they were improbable or because of police action or clerical repression. Sometimes, cases also collapsed because something in the circumstances or the meaning of the apparitions had changed. Often, the phenomena would continue to occur unofficially and locally. In a few rare instances such as Lourdes, there would be

67 'Vigilance de l'église', *Bulletin du diocèse de Reims*, 1876, 667. See, as well, *Le Temps*, 12 March 1877, 2 and *La semaine religieuse du diocèse de Rouen*, 25 December 1875, 1284.

68 Péladan, *(Suite à Dernier mot des Prophéties)*, 19.

69 Ibid., 18.

70 Daurelle, *Les évènements de Fontet d'après les principes de St Thomas*; 'Informations', *Le XIXème siècle*, 26 December 1878, 2.

71 Péladan, *Dernier mot des prophéties*, 13, 145-146. See, as well, Id., *(Suite à Dernier mot des Prophéties)*.

a third stage in which the apparitions would be approved by the Church and become part of the official cult. It is those cases that have mostly attracted the attention of historians to date, Blackbourn notes.[72]

As a visionary, Bergadieu followed the first two stages as outlined by Blackbourn exactly: an initial event, a number of enthusiastic followers, the rapid development of a pilgrimage tradition, the cautious – and at times not so cautious – interest of members of the clergy, and the openness of some in the medical community transformed a local sensation into a possible national phenomenon. For a while, it did appear like Fontet could become the site of a major pilgrimage tradition with all the commercial and touristic interest this could imply for the region and its inhabitants. After all, the phenomena were promising. Bergadieu appeared sincere in her belief in the apparitions and the prophecies she relayed. She did not shy away from visitors, and many were allowed into her bedroom. She was said to like physicians and, to some extent, even welcomed their testing. Her trances were declared real by many witnesses. Observers mentioned that her stigmata were barely noticeable, but her experience of pains of crucifixion appeared to be genuine. The messages pleased both the local community and the country's Legitimists (who, in 1873, were expecting the monarchy to be restored fairly rapidly). As the months passed and with the looming deadline fast approaching, however, doubts began to surface. By 1875, many had lost faith; and with the archbishop of Bordeaux forbidding the clergy from visiting the farm in Fontet and preventing Bergadieu from receiving pilgrims, the phenomena that had so rapidly made the town famous gradually disappeared from the press.

In their work on Marian apparitions, Joachim Bouflet and Philippe Boutry call the period between 1871 and 1917 the time for the apparitions of the *temps mauvais* (bad times). 'Bad times' for the Catholic Church weakened by nationalist movements in Italy, the *Kulturkampf* in Germany, anticlerical trends in France, and rising liberal ideals around Europe. 'Bad times' also for the apparitions themselves, which were now scrutinized by a Church worried about the subversive potential of some these claims.[73] After all, while Maximin Giraud and Mélanie Calvat, the two young visionaries from La Salette, had failed to convince some of the local clergy of their claims, their visions managed to become part of the official cult. Still they continued to create problems for the Church, Mélanie in particular. Her secret, circulated in manuscript throughout the 1860s, was critical of the French clergy and linked the period's political drama to a fight between Christ and Satan.[74] Marie Bergadieu belonged to

72 Blackbourn, *Marpingen*, 6.

73 Bouflet and Boutry, *Un signe dans le ciel*, 165.

74 Mélanie's secret was finally published in 1879. Kaufman, *Consuming Visions*, 21, 24, 26; Kselman, *Miracles and Prophecies*, 62-68, 136-137, and Zimdars-Swartz, *Encountering Mary*, 165-189.

this world in which many in the Church viewed this proliferation of apparitions and prophecies – a number of them apocalyptic – with concern.

What can the story of Bergadieu tell historians? At the very least, it can provide additional evidence of the popularity of Marian apparitions and royalist prophecies in the early years of the Third Republic. Beyond this, it can offer further confirmation of the prudence with which both physicians and many in the Church treated such cases. The story of how Bergadieu's initial and continuing claims were presented, understood, and shaped for a period of a little over two years suggests ways in which a visionary could be seen as genuine even as meanings and explanations about her changed. As her phenomena shifted from apparitions and prophecies to trance, pains of crucifixion, stigmata, and the materialization of the communion wafer, Bergadieu's story was never one of ridicule and derision. Rather, it was one where faith, anxieties, and hope met in a religious and political context that allowed many for a time to consider the possibility that Mary was appearing to a farmer's wife, that monarchy would soon return to France, and that a small town close to Bordeaux would become the next Lourdes.

MEDICAL AND MYSTICAL OPINION IN BRITISH CATHOLICISM

THE CONTENTIOUS CASE OF TERESA HIGGINSON

MARY HEIMANN

Teresa Higginson and her contemporaries

On Good Friday 1874, two years after the highly publicised case of Belgian stigmatic Louise Lateau and a year after Dr Imbert-Gourbeyre brought out his encyclopaedic *Les Stigmatisées* (Paris, 1873), an English Catholic schoolteacher named Teresa Higginson was found lying on her bed in the northern English town of Wigan in the pose of a crucified victim, her hands and feet showing signs of having bled.[1] Higginson's roommate sent for the local Catholic priest, Fr Thomas Wells, who said that he 'did not know what was the matter for her' and told her to 'run for the doctor'.[2] Dr Hart, equally nonplussed, could only comment that the thirty-year-old woman seemed 'extremely weak'.[3]

1 Ryland's notes, Good Friday 1874, in Kerr, *Teresa Helena Higginson: Servant of God, the Spouse of the Crucified*, 78. The first few pages of the present chapter are taken largely from my recent article 'Mysticism in Bootle'. Despite extensive searches, it has proved impossible to find the original collection of letters to, from and about Teresa Higginson, which was first published by O'Sullivan as *Teresa Higginson, the servant of God, school teacher* (London, 1924). This was reprinted with additional letters by Cecil Kerr in 1927, and in an abridged version, as *Teresa Helena Higginson, School Teacher and Mystic*, in 1928. Selected letters were reissued, as a pamphlet, in Honnor, *Appreciations of Teresa Helena Higginson* (1986), and most recently in Whittington-Egan, *The Devil in Bootle* (2010). Published versions of Teresa Higginson's letters are the ones cited throughout the present chapter.

2 Ryland's notes, Good Friday 1874 as reproduced in Kerr, *Teresa Helena Higginson: Servant of God, the Spouse of the Crucified*, 78.

3 Ryland's notes, in Kerr, *Teresa Helena Higginson*, 50, 78.

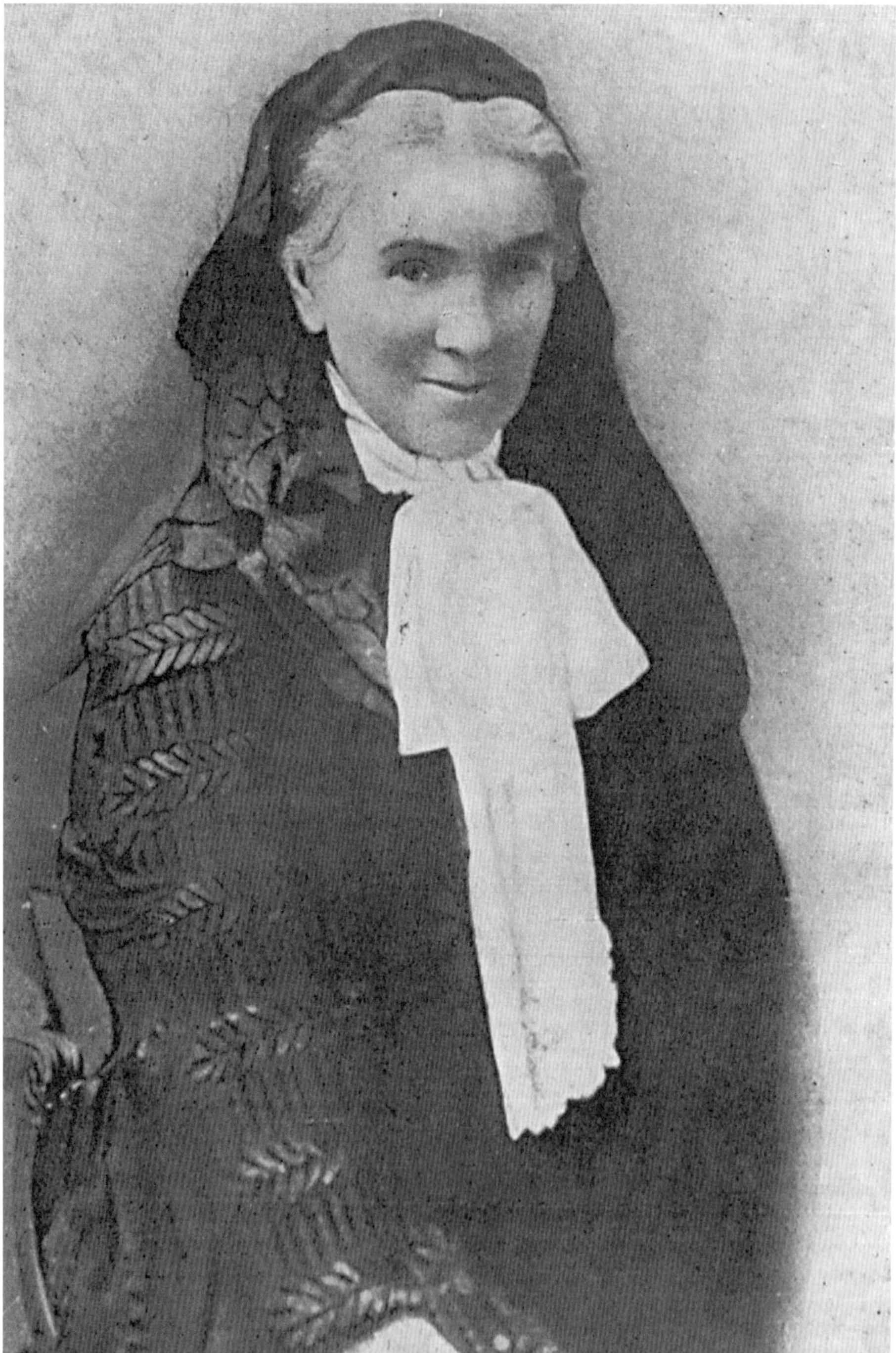

Teresa Higginson.
[*Cecil Kerr.* Thérésa-Héléna Higginson, servante de Dieu, épouse du crucifié]

It was not the first time that this particular teacher at St Mary's Catholic school in Wigan had brought attention to herself. A colleague who shared Teresa Higginson's room – and, indeed, bed – reported hearing strange shrieks, footsteps, knocking, the sound of a person attempting to speak while held by the throat, and 'a rushing noise as if animals were in the room'.[4] Once, she went into their shared room to find the bed charred and smoking, as if someone had set it alight, and Teresa Higginson lying on the floor next to a broken holy water stoup and bottle.[5]

Although neither her priest nor her doctor could account for her strange behaviour, Teresa Higginson evidently had some fairly well developed ideas as to what was going on. As she later explained to a different, more sympathetic, priest than Fr Wells: 'several times when I awoke I perceived a smell of something burning, and the house being filled with smoke and brimstone, I thought surely the house was on fire... other times I saw the whole bed and room full of flames and heard the crackling and I am afraid in this case I proved a coward, for I was frightened more than I can tell at first for there was no holy water: the Devil threw something against the bottle and broke it'.[6] Although some later enthusiasts took Higginson's alleged 'wrangles' with the Devil seriously, at the time Fr. Thomas Wells was less impressed. To Teresa Higginson's explanation that whenever she tried to get up in the night to pray 'the Devil used to beat and ill use the body and spit horrible filth upon me in the face and eyes', the priest responded that he thought she 'had a very fertile imagination'.[7] When the teacher's diabolical 'wrangles', so reminiscent of those reported by the *curé d'Ars*, continued, he reasoned with her as with a child: 'Night time is the time to sleep and rest so that you may be able to do your work as duty requires.'[8] When Higginson persisted in getting up throughout the night, Fr Wells eventually 'commanded' that she stay in bed for at least four hours at a stretch, and added that 'if the will was really desirous of being entirely obedient he did not see how [she] could be so continually rising'.[9] Only when this direct order had no effect did he change tack, humouring her and telling her to 'tell the Devil he must not do it again'. Finally, presumably out of sheer weariness, Fr Wells – who had the local Catholic school as well as the church to run – pleaded with her to 'ask our b.[lessed] Lord to change the temptation'.[10]

The appearance of the 'stigmata', or the signs of Christ's wounds, on Teresa Higginson's prone body on the morning of Good Friday 1874 had not come

4 Ryland to Powell, 27 June 1880, in Kerr, *Teresa Helena Higginson*, 65-67.
5 Ibid.
6 Higginson to Snow, 20 June 1880, in Kerr, *Teresa Helena Higginson*, 61.
7 Ibid., 60.
8 Ibid.
9 Ibid.
10 Ibid., 61-62.

entirely out of the blue. Throughout Holy Week, the schoolteacher had been acting out the drama of her own accompaniment of Jesus along the road to Calvary. Teresa's variations on the Stations of the Cross, as she performed them at St Mary's Church in Wigan, included groans, convulsions, low moans and the frequent recoiling as from invisible blows. Susan Ryland, her fellow-teacher, roommate and 'only friend', spoke to Father Wells about them, but he cautioned her not to get involved.[11] Another teacher, Miss Woodward, raised the matter with her confessor, Father Gradwell SJ. The Jesuit cautiously suggested that she 'take notes of what occurred'.[12] Misses Woodland and Ryland accordingly took turns, for all the world like empirical experimenters, 'to watch and [write] down exactly what they witnessed'.[13] This consisted of seeing Teresa Higginson re-enact, in church, the drama of Christ's Passion. Although ostensibly cast in the role of witness, Teresa tended rather to upstage Christ as she begged an invisible Jesus to take the drink offered to him; to lean on her; to let her guide his feet; to think of his mother's feelings. The pantomime, as recorded by the two teachers, was violent, with Teresa recoiling or crying out from invisible blows, begging Christ's tormentors to 'rend' his clothes less roughly or to lay his body down more gently. The performance ended sensationally, with her body going 'prostrate' and 'still as death' as she continued to imitate Christ through his final agony on the cross.[14]

Although Teresa Higginson's claims cut little ice with Fr Thomas Wells of St Mary's, Wigan, within a few years she had found in nearby Bootle a confessor and spiritual director prepared to believe that the 'visions' and 'pains' she suffered in Holy Week 1874 were mystical 'favours' that presaged greater advances in the spiritual life. As Teresa Higginson explained to her new 'spiritual director', Fr Edward Powell, in a series of letters sent to him from 1878, it was during the latter part of Lent 1874 that Jesus had 'permitted [her] to feel some little of those most cruel torments which He... endured' and 'on the Friday morning in Passion Week [1874], my Lord and my God gave me the marks of His five Sacred Wounds, which I earnestly begged of Him to remove, but to give me an increase if possible of the pain'.[15] During the whole of the following week, she further reported, 'they bled, and Father Wells saw one of them on the Good Friday, after which that disappeared, the others having done so early in the morning; and on several occasions they have re-opened'.[16] Teresa Higginson further explained that she had been granted the privilege of bilocation, actually engaging in missionary work in Africa (where she claimed unparalleled successes in gaining Catholic converts) at the precise moment that

11 Kerr, *Teresa Helena Higginson*, 72.
12 Ibid.
13 Ibid.
14 Ibid., 75.
15 Higginson to [Powell], 24 July 1879, in O'Sullivan, *Teresa Higginson*, 96.
16 Ibid.

eyewitnesses said that she was seated at the dinner table in her lodgings in Wigan.[17]

Six years after receiving the stigmata, Teresa Higginson announced that she had been chosen as the 'spouse of the crucified' in a mystical union that intimately united her to Jesus, allowing her to bear some of the consequences of human sin through her own suffering and enabling her to act as a conduit between the natural and the supernatural worlds.[18] Fresh visions gave her insight into, and then instructed her to spread, a hitherto unknown devotion to the 'Sacred Head' of Jesus.[19] The novel devotion, which was evidently meant to complement and complete existing devotions to the Sacred Heart of Jesus, stressed the importance of the divine wisdom in correcting the intellectual pretensions of Teresa Higginson's own nineteenth century which, as she put it, too often set 'its paltry human sciences against the eternal wisdom of God'.[20] Just as the Sacred Heart was understood to be the focal point for the contemplation of Christ's mercy, compassion and suffering, so the Sacred Head was to be honoured as the seat of divine wisdom, infinite intelligence and the will of God.

Teresa Higginson was not alone in the 1870s and 1880s in claiming diabolical wrangles, bilocation, the stigmata or even mystical espousals: all of these distinctive phenomena from medieval lives of the saints experienced a sharp revival during the latter part of the nineteenth century. Controversies surrounding many contemporary cases involving alleged physical manifestations of mysticism, most of which were widely reported and discussed in medical and psychological as well as in theological and ecclesiastical journals and also in local Church newspapers, were becoming as well-known among Catholics in Britain as on the European continent.[21]

Clerical and lay Catholics living in rural Lancashire and the outskirts of Liverpool in the last quarter of the nineteenth century read and heard sensational reports of contemporary mystics and stigmatics living across the English Channel. They also knew that a rival, purportedly 'scientific', explanatory framework existed to account for mystical phenomena associated with allegedly suggestible Catholic women: the gendered category of 'hysteria'. Susan Ryland, Teresa Higginson's roommate, recalled how 'during the early part of 1874, there was something in the paper about Louise Lateaux [*sic*] in France [*sic*] being in ecstasy every Friday and we passed the remark (I mean Miss Woodward and I) "That is nothing in this house. It is a daily occurrence here",

17 Higginson to [Powell], Feast of the Circumcision 1881, and 2 January 1882, in O'Sullivan, *Teresa Higginson*, 81-92 and in Kerr, *Teresa Helena Higginson*, 355-359.

18 Higginson to [Powell], 3 May 1880, in O'Sullivan, *Teresa Higginson*, 129-132.

19 Higginson to [Powell], 22 June 1879, in O'Sullivan, *Teresa Higginson*, 73-78.

20 Higginson to [Powell], 26 August 1879, in O'Sullivan, *Teresa Higginson*, 78-80.

21 See Imbert-Gourbeyre, *Les Stigmatisées*; Jacobi, *Die Stigmatisierten*; Summers, *The Physical Phenomena of Mysticism* and Thurston, *The Physical Phenomena of Mysticism*.

which it was at that time'.[22] Another teacher remembered how there were days when Teresa Higginson 'literally lived on the Holy Communion and poor Miss Ryland had to half carry her to the altar rails every day. I used to pity the latter, she was a real slave to her.'[23] The same witness recalled how 'one Good Friday when very prostrate and in bed, she spent the day crying and craving the Holy Communion. Of course the confessor paid no attention to her that day but the next she received and was alright [sic] again on the Sunday. Some priests did not believe her and said it was all hysteria.'[24]

Misses Ryland and Woodward, Teresa Higginson's fellow-teachers and housemates, appeared to have accepted the supernatural and magical in their daily lives without difficulty, hardly blinking at the 'miraculous' appearance of new firewood, soap and a key as they went about their business. They mentioned with perfect nonchalance, for example, such claims as that Teresa Higginson could ignite or quench fires by making the sign of the cross over them. They were apparently unprepared to believe that she was mentally ill, leaving it to two local curates to describe her as 'mentally deficient' and 'not fit to be in church'.[25] Nor did they treat her as a saint. Although one might suppose that her re-enactment before their very eyes of scenes from well-thumbed Lives of the saints might have prompted some veneration, or at the very least excitement, they seem to have accepted this behaviour with complacency except when afraid for her physical safety. Fr Wells, on the other hand, was not only unimpressed by her mystical claims, but on at least one occasion drove her out of church in front of everyone. When, claims that Teresa Higginson lived on communion wafers notwithstanding, she was discovered to be eating in secret, she was called a 'lying hypocrite'. Only later was it explained that she was sometimes 'impersonated' by the devil.

Although retrospectively held up as a model Catholic schoolteacher, Teresa Higginson's behaviour was generally considered by her peers to be deviant. In 1876, she was sacked from a teaching job at St Alban's, Liscard. In 1879, she was forced to leave a Jesuit mission school in Sabden, near Clitheroe, 'on account of illness'.[26] In 1877 or 1878 a fellow-lodger accused her of stealing £100; although the money mysteriously reappeared after the police were called, the other residents demanded that she move out.[27] Further accusations in 1879, this time of drunkenness and unseemly behaviour, led to an enquiry being launched by Bishop O'Reilly of Liverpool. He eventually revealed his judgement on the matter by ordering Fr Edward Powell, the first priest to be

22 Kerr, *Teresa Helena Higginson*, 51; Heimann, 'Higginson, Teresa Helena'.

23 As reproduced in Thurston, 'Hagiography: Past and Present', *The Tablet*, 20 November 1937, 684.

24 As reproduced in Ibid., 684.

25 Kerr, *Teresa Helena Higginson*, 183.

26 Lea to Higginson (1879), in Kerr, *Teresa Helena Higginson*, 89.

27 Higginson to Powell (1879), in Kerr, *Teresa Helena Higginson*, 86-87, 94.

sympathetic to her mystical claims, to stop acting as Teresa Higginson's spiritual director.[28] Fr Hall, a Benedictine who was brought in to advise the bishop, pronounced Fr Powell to have been 'duped' by a combination of what he termed 'hysteria' and 'delusion'.[29]

Fr. Edward Powell, although removed as parish priest of St Alexander's Bootle in 1883, nevertheless continued to take an interest in Teresa Higginson's case, and wrote to Fr Bertrand Wilberforce, for an 'expert' opinion on the supernatural experiences that she continued to report. When Fr Bertrand Wilberforce, a Dominican father steeped in the literature of Catholic mysticism and the theology of St Thomas Aquinas, responded to Fr Edward Powell's request for a second opinion on the soul in his care, it was to endorse Teresa Higginson's claims as exactly matching the experiences of a number of canonised saints of the Church. Acknowledging that her devotion to the Sacred Head of Jesus might 'in a certain sense... be called a *new* devotion' he nevertheless judged it to be theologically sound since, as he pointed out, it bore 'a striking analogy to the devotion in honour of the Sacred Heart' and could be defended on the same grounds.[30] Above all, it seemed to meet the more stringent qualification of being a particularly fitting devotion, both in itself and in the timing of its revelation. As Wilberforce argued:

> There is a particular fitness in this devotion to the age in which we live. In order to suit a particular time, a devotion ought to meet the special dangers of the day, supplying an antidote to prevalent spiritual diseases. Now the spirit of this age is evidently one of spiritual rebellion. The human mind intoxicated by modern scientific discoveries is inclined to cast off all restraint and to refuse any longer to remain subject to the sweet yoke of Faith. Rationalism, pure and simple, is the prevailing spirit of the day.[31]

Wilberforce, while admitting that it might be both 'presumptuous' and 'delicate' to pronounce on the character of a soul of a person he had never met, nevertheless found it difficult to moderate his enthusiasm. 'Everything', as he put it, 'that has come to my knowledge, through her letters and accounts given to me by her confessor of her acts and dispositions' all 'lead me to conclude, not only that she is in a high degree of holiness, but also that her mind is wonderfully illuminated by the Light of God.'[32] Systematically combing through Teresa Higginson's letters for evidence of the four traditional virtues associated with sanctity – humility, patience, obedience and mortification –

28 Ibid., 92.
29 Powell to [John Placid] Hall, September 1883, in Kerr, *Teresa Helena Higginson*, 169-170.
30 Wilberforce to Powell, 9 November 1882, Appendix A in Kerr, *Teresa Helena Higginson*, 345-346.
31 Ibid., 348.
32 Ibid., 349.

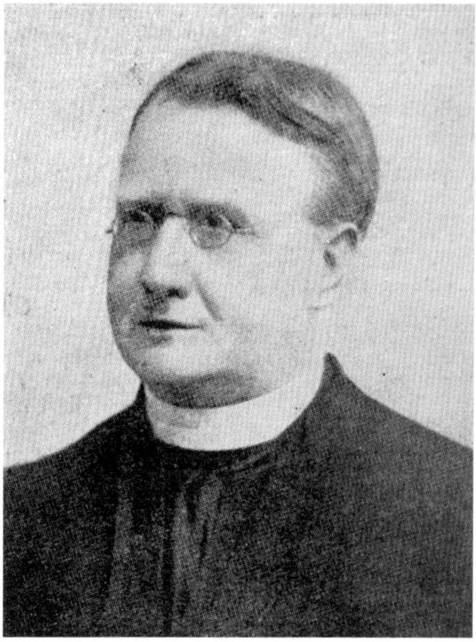

Edward Powell.
[Une grande inconnue ou, Les merveilles d'une simple vie: Teresa Higginson (1844-1905), 32]

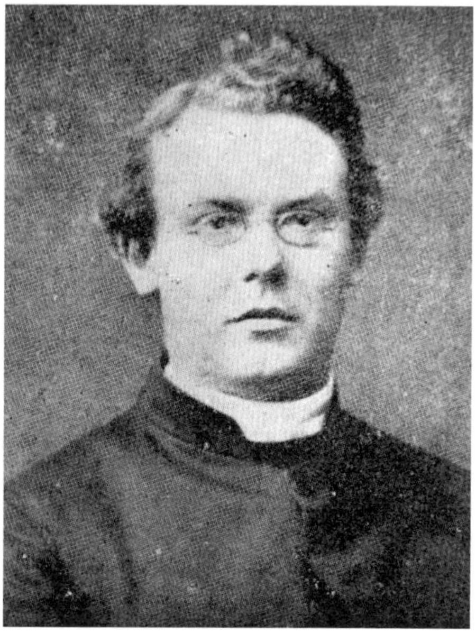

Alfred Snow.
[Une grande inconnue ou, Les merveilles d'une simple vie: Teresa Higginson (1844-1905), 57]

Wilberforce found that she passed all tests with flying colours. In judging Teresa Higginson's humility, he was particularly impressed that 'she thoroughly despises herself, is truly anxious to be despised by others, is free from that self-will which would make her desirous to guide herself instead of submitting to others' and has a 'fear of delusion, yet with confidence in God: is anxious that divine favours should remain hidden, yet mentions them with simplicity under obedience'.[33] Her patience under what he saw as 'the pressure of extreme mental and bodily suffering' Wilberforce found 'heroic', particularly as she not only 'endure[d] these things without repining, but display[ed] an ardent thirst for more numerous and more painful afflictions, in order to unite her soul to Christ crucified'.[34] The testimony of Teresa Higginson's confessor, Fr Edward Powell, that his penitent was immediately willing to cease performing 'any penance or exercise without agitation of mind when commanded' to do so satisfied Fr Wilberforce that she met the requirements of obedience, while her evident self-loathing and pattern of self-harm suggested to him an exemplary 'mortification' of the senses and the successful extinction of self-will.

In 1883, Fr (later Canon) Alfred Snow took over from Fr Edward Powell as Teresa Higginson's 'spiritual director'. Snow proved to be not only a sympa-

33 Wilberforce to Powell, 9 November 1882, Appendix A in Kerr, *Teresa Helena Higginson*, 350.
34 Ibid.

thetic confidant and confessor but also an enthusiastic champion who sought actively to 'prepare' her to receive the 'mystical espousals', the closest possible union of the soul with God. In 1887, after several moves, changes of job and a number of undiagnosed illnesses, and having already claimed to have received miraculous communions and had a vision in which Jesus gave her a ring of thorns and a cross as a token of his betrothal, Teresa Higginson's experiences duly culminated in the final mystical union of 'espousals', which purportedly took place in her lodgings at 53 Lowergate, Clitheroe.

As Teresa Higginson later explained to Fr Alfred Snow, on the night of 23 October 1887 'my divine Spouse spoke to my soul, and said He would now fulfil the promise He had made to me so often and present me to the adorable Trinity and unite Himself to me in the presence of the whole court of heaven.' He then said:

> 'Arise, my beloved, that I may glorify the triune God in unity and espouse thee in their adorable presence.' And turning then to His blessed Mother, He gave me to her as her daughter, and Mary, taking hold of my hand, gave it to Jesus, and He withdrew the ring that he had before placed upon it and then replaced it on the same finger, saying 'I espouse thee in the name and in the presence of the uncreated Trinity and in the presence of My Immaculate Mother, and I give you to her as a daughter and My spouse for ever.' I was wrapped in the Essence of the eternal Godhead and I heard and saw things which it is not given to man to utter.[35]

Snow's reply to Teresa fully endorsed her supernatural claims. 'I praise and thank our dear Lord exceedingly for His great goodness in bestowing this unspeakable favour upon you,' he wrote, 'and I rejoice with you and congratulate you with all my heart upon your marriage with the Lamb, for that is the name of the degree of union to which in His goodness He has now raised you, and it is the highest union to which any soul can attain upon earth.'[36]

Snow then arranged for Teresa Higginson to go to his sister's Convent of the Sisters of Mercy in Edinburgh so that she could fulfil her desire to spread the Devotion to the Sacred Head to Scotland. Teresa ended up spending 12 years in and around Edinburgh, where she set up a makeshift shrine to the Sacred Head and was later claimed by some nuns to have exhibited the stigmata and received miraculous communions. Others, however, recalled how her repeated attempts to open a box by making the sign of the cross over it finally led an impatient nun to send her to fetch the key instead. Although

35 Kerr, *Teresa Helena Higginson*, abridged edition, 53-54.
36 Snow to Higginson, no date, in Whittington-Egan, *The Devil in Bootle*, 165.

Teresa remained a Tertiary of St Francis until her death, she never entered the order of the Sisters of Mercy.[37]

That Teresa Higginson's revelations were doctrinally compatible with the teachings of the Catholic Church, that she appeared always to submit to authority, and that her pronounced desire to suffer seemed to indicate genuine hatred of self, all made the case for her beatification impossible to reject out of hand. On paper at least, she appeared to meet the traditional criteria for sanctity. But what really seemed to persuade Wilberforce of her sanctity was her detailed knowledge of the mystical life, knowledge that he did not believe could have come her way except by direct experience. 'The person has read no books of mystical theology, even the ordinary spiritual books common among the faithful', he wrote in wonderment, 'yet she described most accurately and in most striking terms how a vision which is neither imaginary nor even intellectual is infused by the action of the Holy Spirit in the centre of the soul itself. It is impossible to avoid the impression that she is speaking from personal experience.'[38] Elsewhere, he stressed that 'the theological way in which this simple and unlearned person [sic] explains the doctrine of the Trinity and Incarnation and speaks of devotion to the Sacred Head is a decided indication of superior illumination'. Aware of the existence of an alternative discourse in which Higginson's revelations might be seen as symptoms of 'hysteria', and acknowledging that 'visions are certainly to be more cautiously received in the case of a woman,' Wilberforce nevertheless concluded that 'this soul has had diabolical visions and has detected them.'[39] Fr Wilberforce found it utterly implausible that a person 'unlearned, [who] has read no books [*sic*], and has lived ever secluded [*sic*]' could have 'invented herself a devotion so admirably suited to the times in which we live'.[40] To paint Teresa Higginson – who in fact lived on the outskirts of the bustling metropolis of Liverpool and was employed to teach Catholic doctrine to schoolchildren – as 'secluded' and 'unlearned' was inaccurate: but it helped to give Teresa Higginson credibility as a saint by bracketing her with other purportedly 'simple', 'rural' and 'untutored' female mystics, among others the rising star Bernadette of Lourdes. To Wilberforce, what persuaded was Teresa Higginson's doctrinal precision and apparently close correspondence to the pattern of the saints. The more extravagantly medieval her behaviour and doctrinally precise her language, the more fittingly she could be seen to represent a touchstone of eternal Catholic truth in the midst of nineteenth-century modernity and scepticism, a timely sign that Catholic obedience and simplicity of faith were worth more than all the science and erudition in the world.

37 Whittington-Egan, *The Devil in Bootle*, 171.
38 Ibid., 351.
39 Ibid., 353.
40 Ibid., 352.

Interlude

For nearly fifteen years after Teresa Higginson's death in 1905, her 'holy life and many virtues' seemed, in the words of Teresa Higginson's first hagiographer, 'to have been forgotten'. Even her 'friends and acquaintances', we are told, 'remained silent, not even feeling inclined to talk about her'.[41] In 1922, however, Alfred Snow died. His correspondence with Teresa Higginson passed to the Benedictine monk Adalbert O'Sullivan, who in 1924 published a 'memoir', including a selection of letters, as *Teresa Higginson, the Servant of God, School Teacher*. This first hagiographical sketch set out Teresa Higginson's claims to mystical visions and revelations, together with her devotion to the 'Sacred Head' of Jesus. It took Teresa Higginson's mystical espousals, stigmata and miraculous communions as factually accurate and endorsed her claims to bilocation. It also wrote with confidence of Teresa Higginson's 'proven efficacy', after death, in interceding for 'some pious souls in their needs'.[42] The Benedictine monk, who clearly believed Teresa Higginson to be a saint, sought above all to promote her as 'a Divine gift to her country, a practical example, showing to others in what real sanctity consists, how it ought to be aimed at and how it can be attained by all'.[43]

A second hagiography of this 'servant of God' was brought out in 1927 by Lady Anne Cecil Kerr, the daughter of the 7th Marquis of Lothian and Lady Anne Fitzalan-Howard, this time in the form of a conventional Victorian 'Life and Letters'.[44] Lady Kerr had met Teresa Higginson, remembered as an old lady in black who gave out holy pictures, when she was a child. She embarked on the biography partly because she was intrigued by her mother Anne's description of watching Teresa Higginson pray, apparently glowing and in a state of rapture, at St Catherine's Convent in Edinburgh.[45] The book sold well and an abridged version followed in 1928. Lady Kerr's biography quickly captured the imagination of local Catholics, Irish, English and Scottish, from Merseyside, Lancashire and Edinburgh, where Teresa had spent most of her life; and created a stir among Catholic schoolteachers, who could equally claim Teresa as one of their own, a patron saint advertising the holiness of their professional calling. Miss Catherine Collins, for example, the headmistress of St George's Roman Catholic village school in Maghull, was – perhaps as early as 1928 and certainly no later than 1931 – already a firm believer in Teresa's 'authenticity as a mystic'. Margaret Griffith, too, the head teacher at a Convent school in Surrey, but who originated from Wigan and was a convert, similarly 'used sometimes to mention, with awe, Teresa Higginson'. A former pupil remembered

41 O'Sullivan, *Teresa Higginson*, 12.
42 Ibid., 13.
43 Ibid., 158.
44 *Catholic Herald*, 15 August 1941, 7.
45 Whittington-Egan, *The Devil in Bootle*, 327-328.

how firmly she had 'believed that Teresa was a chosen soul (chosen to suffer for the sins of the world)'.[46]

The excitement generated by Teresa Higginson's growing reputation came, at least in part, as a result of the comparative rarity in Victorian Britain of the mystical phenomena she claimed to have experienced, particularly the stigmata.[47] With her diverse claims to diabolical wrangles, holy ecstasies, miraculous communions, bilocation, invisible supernatural missionary work, visions, stigmata and mystical espousals, Teresa Higginson held the potential to achieve the combined devotional pull of St Francis of Assisi, Bernadette of Lourdes, the *curé d'Ars*, Louise Lateau, Teresa of Avila, St Margaret Mary Alacoque, and many other canonized saints besides. As the daughter of a 'cradle Catholic' and a Catholic convert who was born in Wales, but who was closely associated with Lancashire, Liverpool and Edinburgh, she could be seen to span the United Kingdom and bridge the gap between old Catholics and new while simultaneously linking Catholics of Irish, Welsh, English and Scottish origins. She was able to appeal simultaneously to Irish, convert and Old Catholic girls and ladies, yet could also be seen to represent a hardworking, underpaid and rapidly expanding army of female Catholic schoolteachers at a time of perceived crisis in Catholic education.[48]

The cause for Teresa Higginson's beatification

The cause for Teresa Higginson's beatification was introduced in 1927 by Archbishop Frederick William Keating of Liverpool. As John Davies has found, it was vigorously promoted in the pages of Liverpool's *The Cathedral Record* and in *The Harvest* in the nearby diocese of Salford. Both local Catholic newspapers included many accounts of 'miracles' attributed to Teresa Higginson's intercession and gave plenty of space to the enthusiastic promotion of her cause by local clergy, both secular and religious.[49] In 1933, Fr Frederick Kershaw, the Ushaw-educated editor of *The Harvest*, brought out the pamphlet *Teresa Helena Higginson: A Short Account of her Life and Letters* at the explicit request of the Salford Teachers' Guild.[50]

The case for Teresa Higginson's beatification was formally presented to the Sacred Congregation of Rites in Rome on 7 December 1933, accompanied by a flurry of pamphlets, hagiographies and devotional tracts, together with

46 Unpublished letter from Florence Julien to the author, 12 March 1990, ff.1;3.

47 Mary Ann Girling, a stigmatic of Protestant background, was a notable exception. See Heimann, 'Mary Ann Girling' and Rose, *The Woman who Claimed to be Christ*.

48 On the crisis in Catholic education see, for example, Tenbus, *English Catholics and the Education of the Poor*, 89-117.

49 Davies, 'Traditional Religion, Popular Piety, or Base Superstition?', 125.

50 Kershaw, *Teresa Helena Higginson*.

continued favourable local Lancashire and Liverpool press in the pages of the *Harvest* and *Cathedral Record*. Most significantly, the Catholic Truth Society of Ireland brought out a 20-page version of Cecil Kerr's *Life* that bore an imprimatur and appeared to imply official Church approval of her sanctity. A Dutch translation of Cecil Kerr's 'official biography' of the 'spouse of the crucified' was published simultaneously in The Hague and Antwerp in the same year and a French edition followed a year and a half later.[51] The cause seemed set to spread in much the same way that the reputation of contemporary French, German, Italian and Belgian mystics had spread. Exact contemporary St Gemma Galgani, for example, who received the stigmata a decade later than Teresa Higginson but died three years before her, was declared venerable in 1931, blessed in 1933, and finally canonized in 1940.

On 8 June 1935, the *Catholic Herald* reported that 'preliminary investigations in connection with the Cause for the Canonization of Teresa Higginson Committee' had concluded with a pilgrimage, organized by the Liverpool Archdiocesan Catholic Teachers' Teresa Higginson Committee, of around 500 people to her graveside at St Winifrede's Church in Neston. Petitions for the cause of Teresa Higginson's beatification were by then claimed to have 'exceeded 100,000' and to been received 'from nearly every country in the world'.[52] By November 1936, 'an inaugural meeting consisting mainly of teachers', was held in the bishop of Liverpool's Cathedral Hall and the principal of St Mary's College 'spoke of the great honour that it would be to the Catholic body of teachers if the first person to be raised to the altars of the Church since the Reformation should be one of their own profession – "a Teacher Saint"'.[53]

The Irish Catholic Truth Society pamphlet brought the story of Teresa Higginson within reach of anyone who looked through the information leaflets, prayer-cards and requests for donations to be found at the back of any parish church. One Anglican clergyman was so shocked to find that an organization calling itself 'the Catholic Truth Society' would countenance such claptrap that he wrote to *The Modern Churchman* in May 1936 to declare it 'clear that this woman was a pathological case and, like so many religious neurotics, the victim of hallucinations'. While he conceded that Teresa Higginson might faithfully have imitated 'the experiences of the saints', what she spouted was not 'spiritual wisdom' but 'trash worthy of a spiritualistic séance'. The 'Higginson pamphlet', he concluded disdainfully, 'is the type of literature considered quite suitable by the Jesuits in Manchester as spiritual pabulum for the faithful. The stuff is nonsense, but the right kind of nonsense, and the Jesuit

51 Kerr, *Teresa Helena Higginson: de bruid van den gekruisigde*; Id., *Thérésa-Héléna Higginson, servant de Dieu épouse du crucifié*.

52 *Catholic Herald*, 8 June 1935, 15.

53 'A Teacher Saint', *Catholic Herald*, 27 November 1936, 14.

Fathers collect the public's tuppences by retailing it at the Church of the Holy Name.'[54]

Publicity surrounding the cause for Teresa Higginson's beatification, which included increasingly extravagant claims of miraculous intercessions, matched a parallel French campaign for devotions to the 'Holy Face' that caused considerable embarrassment to those French Catholic clergy who were seeking to distance themselves from reliance on the physical manifestations of mysticism.[55] Indeed, one of Teresa Higginson's greatest champions proved to be Mère Guélin, foundress of the Servants of Jesus-Wisdom at Cagnotte in the Landes district of France and editor of the bi-monthly devotional bulletin *Sagesse*. Guélin made many references to Teresa Higginson in her devotional writings, dedicated a pamphlet to her, and sought to spread the Devotion to the Sacred Head. This sort of thing was every bit as embarrassing to self-consciously enlightened members of the English Catholic community as to their 'rationalist' French counterparts.

In March 1937, two damning French Catholic accounts of Teresa Higginson were reprinted in *The Clergy Review*, the 'progressive' new journal for Catholic priests that had been founded in 1931. The first negative remark came through a review of a special volume of *Études Carmélitaines* dedicated to 'the pressing problem of stigmatization' which it discussed from 'every angle, historical, physiological, psychological, psychiatric and theological' and which included a dismissive footnote about Teresa Higginson.[56] The second, more focussed critique, came in a review of the 1935 French edition of Cecil Kerr's 'official' biography of Teresa Higginson. This rejected the case for the English stigmatic's beatification with the damning indictment that all evidence rested on 'a woman's testimony' and, moreover, one with a 'sickly' character.[57] According to the report in *The Clergy Review*, Teresa Higginson's education 'predisposed her to become mystical' whereas 'her phenomena, which she herself first observed, were seen by others because they were psychically dominated; the

54 Hardwick in *The Modern Churchman* (May 1936), as reproduced in Whittington-Egan, *The Devil in Bootle*, 259-260.

55 *Études Carmélitaines* under the editorship of Bruno de Jésus-Marie, as Agnès Desmazières has found, was at the forefront of a new movement to promote a distinctive Catholic psychology in answer to atheistic alternatives. See Desmazières, *L'Inconscient au paradis*, 64-66. Some influential contemporary English Catholic clergy and laity similarly sought to promote Catholic solidarity among medics, first through the Catholic Medical Guild. In 1935, as discussed below in the text, a new Catholic Psychological Society was set up.

56 J. Cartmell, 'Notes on Recent Work. Ascetical and Mystical Theology', *The Clergy Review*, 13 (1937) 2, 96.

57 M. Claeys Boúúaert, 'C. Kerr, *Theresia Helena Higginson ou la vie merveilleuse d'une institutrice libre anglaise*, tr par V. Billé', *Nouvelle Revue Théologique*, 63 (1936) 9, 1088. The Kerr biography was published in French in 1935. The special issue was published in Paris by Desclée de Brouwer et Cie.

atmosphere around her was pregnant with hallucinations'.[58] Particularly disturbing, in *The Clergy Review*'s estimation, was 'the excuse offered by Teresa when certain accusations were made against her that the devil had personated her'. Neither her claims to stigmata nor to 'prolonged fast', it noted, had been 'rigorously checked' by independent witnesses. Finally, although the 'detailed findings' of the episcopal enquiry that had looked into her case were not known, the bishop had ultimately found against her. It seemed especially telling that the 'two priests who took part in the enquiry ceased to believe in the phenomena' once all the available evidence was brought to light.[59]

In May 1937, the archbishops and bishops of Scotland threw their weight behind the northern schoolteachers and Catholic Truth Society of Ireland, directly petitioning Rome for the beatification of Teresa Higginson on the grounds that since she had spent 'nearly 12 years with us and was fond of our country' (i.e. Scotland, as opposed to the United Kingdom), the archbishop and bishops of Scotland were bound to do all they could 'to promote her cause'.[60] This marked the beginning of a veritable battle between Teresa Higginson's North Country champions and her equally tenacious London detractors that was fought out in the pages of *The Tablet* between May 1937 and April 1938. The cause was an appropriate one for *The Tablet*: the urbane English Catholic weekly, previously controlled by successive archbishops of Westminster, had in 1935 been taken over by a group of English Catholic laymen who sought to cater for a cultured Catholic elite as part of their broader mission to integrate Catholics into respectable English society. In 1936 they appointed as editor Douglas Woodruff, an eminent journalist at *The Times* and a Catholic who was married to Lord Acton's granddaughter. Woodruff, who was described at his funeral as 'the Chesterbelloc' of the post-war Church and 'a great Christian gentleman', turned *The Tablet* into a platform for Hilaire Belloc, Evelyn Waugh, Graham Greene, Ronald Knox, Martin D'Arcy, Christopher Dawson and many other Catholic novelists and intellectuals.[61]

In the same year that *The Tablet* was being revamped, a 'group of medical psychologists, clergy and others' met together at Heythrop College to form a new 'Catholic Psychological Society' whose stated aim was to publicize, lecture and otherwise inform Catholics about the new branch of medicine.[62] Hav-

58 J. Cartmell, 'Notes on Recent Work. Ascetical and Mystical Theology', *The Clergy Review*, 13 (1937) 2, 97.

59 Ibid.

60 For the final, typed petition, see Edinburgh, Scottish Catholic Archives, Diocese of Dunkeld, DG/14/19/1: 'In Causa Beatificationis et Canonizationis Teresiae Helenae Higginson' (Archbishop Joseph Andrews to the Holy Father, 1 May 1937), for the handwritten English version, headed 'Rough Translation', see DD/15/30/6.

61 Archbishop Derek Worlock, 'Requiem address for Douglas Woodruff', *The Tablet*, 18 March 1978, 36.

62 'A Catholic Psychological Society', *The Tablet*, 30 November 1935, 23; 'The Catholic Medical Guild', *The Tablet*, 26 October 1935, 18.

ing already expended considerable ink in seeking to discredit the Victorian vogue for spiritualism, self-consciously rational Catholic apologists sought to subject mystical claims to medical scrutiny. 'All that glitters is not gold,' declared the neurologist F.M.R. Walshe, pointedly signing himself as a 'Catholic doctor' in a letter to *The Tablet* published on 8 May 1937. The case of Teresa Higginson, he pleaded, needed to be investigated from a 'psycho-pathological point of view' since, as a 'Catholic doctor' with knowledge of 'the field of nervous disorders', he could see that 'the obviously medical elements in the story, the mysterious illnesses, the swoons and trances, the romancing as to wounds said to have been caused by practices of mortification, and the alleged agonies of pain' were all 'the constituents, clear and unequivocal, of an hysterical illness, nor [was] there any available medical alternative interpretation thereof'.[63] That Dr Walshe's intervention was not dictated by disinterested medical curiosity alone, but also intended to contain the spread of what he considered to be inappropriate expressions of sanctity, can be discerned by his dry comment that 'Lives such as hers are more commonly recorded abroad than in this country, whose spirituality is perhaps more characteristically expressed by the lives of SS. John Fisher and Thomas More than by the bizarre career of this North Country school teacher.'[64]

The sense that the extravagant claims made by and about Teresa Higginson could only bring Catholicism into disrepute, as a credulous set of superstitions, was echoed by other correspondents writing in *The Tablet* who were working hard to move Catholicism out of the 'ghetto' into mainstream, middle-class English life. So-called traditional 'recusant' or 'Old Catholic' Catholicism in England and Scotland prided itself on its sobriety, steadfastness and discretion. In matters of taste, it was supposed to be at the other end of the spectrum from the emotive revivalism spread by religious orders such as the Passionists, Redemptorists, Brompton Oratorians and St Vincent de Paul Society. The elephant in the room was the 'vulgar piety' of stereotypical Irish Catholic working-class immigrants, whose supposed tendency towards 'superstition' was not only the bane of many English Catholic clergy, but felt by some socially respectable Catholics to make their religion ridiculous in the eyes of non-Catholics.[65]

The 1930s was an important period of growth in respectability for the English Catholic community. Campion Hall in Oxford and the nearby Jesuit College at Heythrop were establishing themselves, and Jesuit confessors – most notably the Harrow and Oxford-educated Jesuit Cyril Charles (C.C.) Martindale, himself a convert to Catholicism – were proving skilled at attracting converts of the calibre of Graham Greene, Muriel Spark and Evelyn Waugh.

63 Walshe, 'Teresa Higginson', *The Tablet*, 8 May 1937, 666.
64 Ibid., 665.
65 Gilley, 'Vulgar Piety and the Brompton Oratory'.

A distinctive blend of light-hearted wit, love of logic, and underlying moral earnestness could be felt in the works of English Catholics as various as G.K. Chesterton and Ronald Knox. Catholic Social Action was also booming, and the Catholic Workers' College, later renamed Plater College, was making its way in Oxford. At the same time that George Orwell was writing his *The Road to Wigan Pier*, Catholicism was managing to recruit from both sides of an increasingly bitter class war, from the political Left as well as the political Right. To those who wished to see English Catholics fully integrated into the Anglican-dominated establishment, the cause for Teresa Higginson's beatification could hardly have come at a more awkward time.

In mid-October 1937, at the height of the *Tablet* dispute, over 700 people turned up to a rally in Clapham in 'support' of Teresa Higginson that was organized by the London Teachers Committee. The rally boasted 11 parish rectors and 2 provincials and was favourably covered by the *Catholic Herald*.[66] The prominent Jesuit scholar Herbert Thurston, whose reputation for scepticism made him the ideal investigator of bogus claims of the supernatural and paranormal, and whose interests stretched to poltergeists, spiritualists and mediums as well as to mystics,[67] sprang into action. Unearthing passages from letters that had been omitted in Cecil Kerr's *Life*, and which shed less flattering light on Teresa Higginson, Thurston presented her as a demanding neurotic and attention-seeking drain on her fellow-teachers. The Farm Street scholar not only cast doubt on Cecil Kerr's reliability and integrity as a biographer, but claimed to see in Teresa Higginson 'that strong egotism which is so integral a part of the symptom-complex of hysteria: a symptom-complex which figures so largely and so intimately in the life of Miss Higginson, and lends this life so pathological a complexion in the eyes of any informed and critical reader'.[68] Although medicalized terms and unflattering testimonies might hurt the innocent piety of Higginson's many 'North Country' champions, Thurston insisted that 'nothing less than a fastidious regard for accuracy and candour' was due to the 'trusting audiences' of hagiographies, all the more so since 'a cause that goes to Rome from this country carries with it, in a sense, the good name of English Catholicism'.[69]

Champions of the cause for Teresa Higginson's beatification quickly came forward to defend her reputation. One letter to *The Tablet*, signed 'Teacher's Friend', claimed to see in Thurston's letter 'an undercurrent of envy' and asked sarcastically whether St Peter, 'a tough old fisherman' yet who was said

66 *Catholic Herald*, 15 October 1937, accessed 4 September 2013 at <http://archive.catholicherald.co.uk/article/15th-october-1937/1>. The provincials were of the Oblates of St Charles and the Salesians.
67 Heimann, 'Herbert Henry Charles Thurston'.
68 Thurston, 'Hagiography: Past and Present', *The Tablet*, 20 November 1937, 684.
69 Ibid.

in the Gospel to have 'wept bitterly' ought similarly to be 'considered an egoist, indulging in a symptom-complex of hysteria? Nevertheless he has been canonized. I wonder how St Mary Magdalen and St Monica got away with it?'[70] Thomas S. Kelly, the brother of the priest at St Alexander's, Bootle, argued that although it might 'be difficult to prove that these incidents of bilocation occurred' it would be 'equally difficult to prove that they did not'.[71] A 'psychologist', he crushingly concluded, is 'of course, quite at liberty to look upon the mystic experiences of Teresa as "mental aberrations"', but would need to reconcile allegations of mental illness with 'her life-long reputation for perfect truthfulness and remarkable commonsense [sic]'.[72] 'Simplicity' of faith, argued another defender, was a surer guide than 'modern scepticism' to discerning holiness.[73]

The stakes were rising. The normally harmless, even commendable, 'simple piety' of uneducated Catholics, including many Irish-born Liverpool, Birmingham, London and Lancashire Catholics, was beginning to seem less benign to the English Catholic intelligentsia archetypically represented by the Jesuits of Farm Street in London. 'Let us remember', warned Thurston, that if Teresa Higginson 'should be beatified, she will be the first English non-martyr to be raised to the altars of the Church for more than six hundred years. Such an event is likely to attract a certain amount of notice even in the Anglican and secular Press.'[74] Is it too much, he asked, 'that if our ideals of holiness are to be subjected to the criticism of our non-Catholic fellow countrymen, we should like to be represented by a type of sanctity somewhat less extravagant than that revealed in the story of Teresa Higginson?'[75] An alarmed English Catholic laywoman was similarly 'filled with dismay' at the thought 'that Teresa Higginson, a pious woman no doubt, but exhibiting every symptom of neurotic disorder, should be presented to the world as the nearest approach to the ideal of sanctity which England has produced in six hundred years'.[76]

The problem was not just that Teresa Higginson was peculiar and might have been mad. According to J.S. Cammack, SJ, Professor of Moral Philosophy at Heythrop College, one of the most serious contemporary dangers to faith consisted in taking purely 'physiological and materialistic factors as an adequate explanation of mental deviations in character'.[77] Teresa Higginson's champions were, in his view 'confusing essential sanctity and the accidental

70 'Teacher's friend', Letter to the Editor, *The Tablet*, 11 December 1937, 803.
71 Kelly, Letter to the Editor, *The Tablet*, 25 December 1937, 886.
72 Ibid.
73 'A Colonial Reader', Letter to the Editor, *The Tablet*, 11 December 1937, 803.
74 Thurston, 'Beatification', *The Tablet*, 15 January 1938, 73.
75 Ibid.
76 M. Catherine Ashburnham, 'Letter to the Editor', *The Tablet*, 29 January 1938, 151.
77 Cammack, *Moral Problems of Mental Defect*. See also book review by F. Emory Lyon in the *Journal of Criminal Law and Criminology*, 30 (1940), 976-978.

phenomena which may accompany it'.[78] Even, as he put it, 'if it were proved that the startling mystical phenomena in Teresa's life were due to some form of hysteria' this would be 'no obstacle to her beatification if it were proved that her life showed the exercise of the theological and moral virtues in an heroic degree'.[79] C.C. Martindale, S.J., agreed, pointing out that 'words like "neurotic", "hysterical" have not yet found a definition in which all agree: but none of them (I think) need connote anything "moral" at all. We can, then, imagine a neurotic, anaemic, or hysterical saint'.[80] The problem that the Jesuits had identified was this: sanctity did not depend on extravagant mystical phenomena; but it did depend on heroic virtue. 'There is, I suppose there *can* be, no evidence for any of Miss Higginson's strange experiences save her *ipsa dixi*', Martindale considered; 'nor is there evidence that her director (the first thing that an ecstatic seeks), though able to discern virtue, was skilled too in abnormal psychology (unconscious fraud included)'.[81] All the more rigorously must the public be safeguarded 'from thinking for a moment that her virtue, however heroic, consisted in, even issued into, or maybe had anything at all to do with, those experiences, alleged by her, which are bound so seriously to disconcert so many'.[82] An Italian professor of dogmatic theology riposted that this seemed to mean that 'God is acceptable only when He presents Himself dressed in the fashion of a gentleman according to current tests'.[83]

As one side in the debate continued to play the supernaturalist card, the other resorted increasingly to that of scientific authority. 'As doctors', declared Dr Walshe, 'we are vividly aware, to a degree impossible to a non-medical student' that 'the manifestations of a psychoneurosis may assume the outward expressions of sanctity and produce a caricature of it'.[84] It was not, he declared pointedly, 'the critics' of Teresa Higginson who were 'the mystagogues'.[85] Stigmatics, 'with the honourable exception of St Francis of Assisi', were generally 'hysterics' and 'psychologically ill liars' who 'simulated nonexistent symptoms'.[86] Dr Letitia Fairfield of Gray's Inn, seizing upon the 'important admission' that 'no medical opinion' had been sought by those engaged in the canonization process,[87] wondered how the Commission could possibly 'know the facts really *were* facts unless they went beyond mere "collection", a task for which a mixed tribunal of solicitors' clerks and shorthand

78 J.S. Cammack, Letter to the Editor, *The Tablet*, 22 January 1938, 118.
79 Ibid.
80 C.C. Martindale, Letter to the Editor, *The Tablet*, 22 January 1938, 119.
81 Ibid.
82 Ibid.
83 E. Campana, Letter to the Editor, *The Tablet*, 22 January 1938, 121.
84 Walshe, Letter to the Editor, *The Tablet*, 29 January 1938, 150.
85 Ibid.
86 Ibid.
87 L. Fairfield, Letter to the Editor, *The Tablet*, 12 February 1938, 213.

typists would have been adequate'.[88] The point did not, she insisted, 'turn on whether or not "preternatural happenings are essential to sanctity" (which no one maintains), but that on a medical view, Teresa's neurotic mentality caused her to allege that such happenings had occurred when, in fact, they had not'.[89] There had already, she judged, been 'a terrifying assumption' in much of *The Tablet* correspondence that 'allegations of fraud, injustice and dishonesty directed against a candidate for beatification are "trivial"'. For her own part, the barrister wished 'very respectfully' to submit 'that the present state of her Cause is an affront to reason and a peril to the Faith'.[90] Walshe concluded his own diatribe by welcoming the 'encouragement' given in an address on psychology 'recently delivered by His Grace the Archbishop of Liverpool, in which he urged Catholics no longer to stand aside from the use of the knowledge provided by modern advances in psychology'.[91]

Although there were some obvious regional, gender, social and economic dimensions to the split between Teresa Higginson's promoters and detractors, such divisions were by no means absolute and do not tell the whole story. When Thurston tried to pass off the movement for Higginson's beatification as limited to 'Catholic schoolteachers as a body', the 'people of Bootle' and 'a considerable number of good Lancashire folk' who were 'very keen about her' and 'would like to have a canonized Saint of their very own', [92] there was not enough space to print all the outraged responses.[93] From Heythrop, where 'about seventy people, just over a third' of the College's male members, signed a petition in Teresa Higginson's favour, J.S. Cammack argued that although 'a clinical picture of a typical psycho-neurotic' could 'be constructed', this could only be done 'by ignoring the contrary indications, selecting the unfavourable facts and interpreting them without using the criteria of mystical and ascetical theology'.[94] Even if Dr Walshe were capable of explaining 'how a complete hysteric could suddenly become, and remain, normal without some form of psychic compensation' or could 'construct a perfectly coherent explanation of a very tricky point in theology',[95] the question might nevertheless remain debatable 'in view of the well-known differences between the various schools of psychological medicine'.[96] Most of all, the Jesuit scholar objected to 'the chiding tone' adopted by those who wished to discredit the Cause, pointing out that 'the opponents of this case are not naughty children airing their un-

88 L. Fairfield, Letter to the Editor, *The Tablet*, 12 February 1938, 213-214.
89 Ibid., 214.
90 Ibid.
91 Walshe, Letter to the Editor, *The Tablet*, 29 January 1938, 150.
92 Thurston, Letter to the Editor, *The Tablet*, 29 January 1938, 151.
93 Letters to the Editor, *The Tablet*, 5 February 1938, 174.
94 Cammack, Letter to the Editor, *The Tablet*, 5 February 1938, 174.
95 Ibid.
96 Ibid.

orthodox views and "presumably in good faith", but experts who genuinely believe that they have a solid case to be exposed for the good of the Church'.[97]

In the face of strong opposition, even from within his own Society of Jesus, to what was criticized as materialist reductionism, Thurston moved away from psychology to textual criticism. He noted that the Irish Catholic Truth Society pamphlet had omitted to include 'all reference to "the curse pronounced against those who shall hinder and despise this devotion (to the Sacred Head)"' who Teresa Higginson had claimed would be '"as an egg that is thrown to the wall; they shall be shattered and become as nought and shall be dried and wither as grass on the house-top"'. Nor, he observed, had the Irish Catholic Truth Society pamphlet included mention of the visits that Teresa claimed to her confessor to have 'been paying for four years together to the tribe of Ja-am-pu-da in Africa, her body presumably remaining the while in Lancashire'.[98] Higginson's so-called 'bilocations', jibed another critic, were 'low grade' even as products of the imagination: 'our school children, were they asked to imagine themselves missioners among blacks, would produce something better than this'.[99]

Walshe followed Thurston's move from neurology to character assassination. Although Teresa Higginson had indeed been a schoolteacher 'it cannot be said she was a model one' since she was 'thoroughly undependable', 'frequently absent', 'forced others to be absent also' and was a 'hindrance to her colleagues'.[100] Fellow teacher Miss Woodward, for example, remembered how annoying it had been to have to put up with Teresa Higginson's constant demands for attention: 'I used to think she ought to exert her will more and not be such a burden on poor Miss Ryland, who got quite worn out, and of course, while she was attending and waiting on her (Miss H.) She was absent from her own school which was then left solely to me: consequently we got into disrepute with the Inspector and I thought this unfair to Miss Ryland.'[101] Similarly, a 'lady who deputized for Teresa at Chudleigh' recalled how Higginson used frequently 'to whip the children' and how the report from the religious inspector was 'so bad that Fr. Dowsett told me he stuck it in the fire' since the children 'just knew scarce anything of their catechism'. Teresa Higginson, Walshe concluded, was a teacher 'whom no Catholic school manager would today dare to employ'.[102]

97 Ibid.
98 Fairfield, Letter to the Editor, *The Tablet*, 12 February 1938, 214.
99 A Vice-Postulator, Letter to the Editor, *The Tablet*, 19 February 1938, 247.
100 Walshe, Letter to the Editor, *The Tablet*, 26 February 1938, 277.
101 As reproduced in H. Thurston, 'Hagiography: Past and Present', *The Tablet*, 20 November 1937, 683. This less flattering portion of an otherwise positive letter was not included in Cecil Kerr's biography.
102 Walshe, Letter to the Editor, *The Tablet*, 26 February 1938, 277.

By this point, Thomas Kelley of Wallasey could stand no more. Declaring *The Tablet* correspondence to have 'gone far enough', he accused the editor of having 'permitted correspondents to sniff at an accepted candidate for Church honours' and to brand her as a liar and a fraud as well as to allow 'critics to sneer at the friends of Teresa, both living and dead'.[103] The 'opinions of untrained minds illumined by faith', he retorted, were 'worth immeasurably more than those of trained minds blinded by prejudice or hampered by the exigencies of a superiority complex'.[104] Were 'nothing more important than the merits of Teresa Higginson' at stake, replied Dr Walshe, Wallasey's pleas to stop the barrage of criticism of the North Country teacher would be valid: what was 'at issue', however, was 'of fundamental importance to English Catholicism: namely, a sound and sane standard of spiritual values'.[105]

Two distinct discourses emerged from *The Tablet* correspondence, each offering a rival vision of how a self-consciously Catholic minority ought to present itself to the surrounding predominantly Protestant, and secularising, world. From one point of view, promoted mainly from Liverpool and Lancashire (where Teresa had the potential to be seen as a local saint), and also by Catholic schoolteachers (the vast majority of whom were women), the cause for her beatification was tied up with a sense, not just of local patriotism, but also of the need to engage intensely with the mystical traditions of Catholic hagiography and to embrace all that made Catholicism distinctive. Letters written by those who favoured Teresa Higgionson's cause tended to be written in explicitly Catholic hagiographical language and to spill over with religious revivalist emotion, gushing with gratitude for her intercession or pointing out her theological virtues in stock religious phrases. They reeked, in short, of the Catholic ghetto.

The timeliness of Teresa Higginson's call to abandon reliance on human intellect and lean instead on the 'Sacred Head' as the 'seat of divine wisdom' was frequently reiterated by Teresa Higginson's advocates, as was the need for a patron saint of Catholic teachers. Our home-grown English Catholic saints, Higginson's supporters seemed to be saying, are just as mystical, miraculous and flamboyant as any to be found in medieval or contemporary Italy, France or Belgium; furthermore, our faith is more pure and authentic, because more humble, faithful and heartfelt, than that of coolly superior English intellectuals. There was a professional and class, as well as a devotional, dimension to this Catholic revivalist ethos, as working-class and lower-middle-class teachers made populist appeals and drew on the methods of the modern pressure-group to gather signatures for petitions and organize mass rallies for the cause. Teresa Higginson's lay supporters further organized tours and pilgrimages to

103 Thomas S. Kelly, Letter to the Editor, *The Tablet*, 19 February 1938, 247.
104 Ibid., 249.
105 Walshe, Letter to the Editor, *The Tablet*, 26 February 1938, 278.

the places she had lived and taught, and to the graveyard where she lay buried; distributed prayer-cards for her cause to be victorious and set up shrines and devotions to the Sacred Head wherever they could. Those that opposed Teresa Higginson's beatification were deeply embarrassed by the oddity of the schoolteacher and her new-fangled devotion, the extravagance of the claims made for her and the credulity which was apparently expected from her biographers and supporters. Above all, they were concerned about the poor impression her case would make on their non-Catholic countrymen, returning them to ridicule and suspicion – to the ghetto – just as they were coming to be accepted in polite society.

Rejection

The case for Teresa Higginson's beatification was formally refused by Rome on 7 December 1938. The Catholic Church's stamp of approval was removed from both the Irish Catholic Truth Society pamphlet, which was withdrawn from circulation, and from her cherished 'Devotion to the Sacred Head'. A radio talk by a Catholic priest from Dublin on the 'Life of Teresa Higginson' was nevertheless broadcast, first in Irish and then in English, fourteen months later, by which point England was at war with Germany (and Ireland was not).[106] This radio talk was peppered with references to Teresa Higginson's likeness to saints Thérèse of Lisieux, the *Curé d'Ars* and Teresa of Avila, as well as to her association with well-known revivalist priests such as Father Faber, Fr Ignatius Spencer and Venerable Dominic Barberi. It further included the names of many local 'witnesses', still living, who could attest to her supposed 'gentleness, her kindness and her wonderful religious teaching'.[107] The broadcast asserted that Teresa Higginson had 'gained her Teaching Certificate in a miraculous way', gained a 'share' in Christ's sufferings and 'even the Sacred Stigmata', and, 'like St John Vianney (the Curé of Ars)', been 'tormented by the devil'. It reproduced the claims that 'Our Lord frequently gave Himself to

106 The talk, entitled 'Teresa Helena Higginson', was broadcast from Dublin by Michael O'Mullin on Radio Eireann on 4 March 1940. It was advertised in the *Catholic Herald* (1 March 1940).

107 Edinburgh, Scottish Catholic Archives, DE/142/Saints-Causes and Pilgrimages/52: Higginson, Michael O'Mullin, 'Teresa Helena Higginson' (unpublished transcript of talk broadcast by Radio Eireann, 4 March 1940), f. 4. Locals who helped O'Mullin during his 'first visit to Neston' in October 1937 included: Mrs Brennan of Exeter Road; Fr Horner of St Alexander's, Bootle; Mr. Annesley, 'who had been to Teresa's grave too'; Miss Flaherty of Burton Road, 'a lady well known to all pilgrims to Neston'. During his second visit, in October 1938, Mrs Helen Lonsdale of Wigan told him 'wonderful stories of Teresa' and 'showed me several letters written by her'; he also spent two evenings 'with Mr Garnett, the lifelong friend of Teresa Higginson' and Miss Arkwright 'whose work for Teresa is known and appreciated from Alaska through America and Europe to Australia and New Zealand'.

her in Holy Communion', that she 'wrote inspired letters on the great Truths of our Church' and that she found 'the closest union with God possible to a soul on earth' through Mystical Marriage. Only the claims to bilocation in order to undertake secret missionary work in Africa for the Ja-am-pu-da tribe appear to have been quietly omitted.

By January 1945, the activities of a 'Teresa Higginson Association' led by Edward Lonsdale of Standish, Wigan and Lawrence Harvey of Neston, Cheshire, had become of sufficient concern to the archbishop of Liverpool for him to declare the association 'inexpedient' and to insist that its leaflets be withdrawn and lectures on the 'Life of Teresa Higginson' cease.[108] Concern at the 'increased activities of these people and of their colleagues' led the archbishop to bring the case to his superior's attention a month later.[109] The activity appears to have been successfully suppressed, since by 1951 it was left to a lone individual, Mrs Bridget McVey, *née* McClusky of Dalkeith, to write a confused letter to the pope that included claims of 'first class evidence' for 'Teresa Higginson the Lancashire stigmatist' on the strength of her own 'bilocation' and visions.[110]

The secular, psychologically-minded mood of Britain in the 'swinging' 1960s and 1970s proved a relatively barren period for the cause of Teresa Higginson, as for other Catholic stigmatics and mystics; but the return to conservative values, local patriotism and religious revivalism from the 1980s, together with a parallel rise of popular interest in alternative spiritualities, the paranormal and the occult, changed the religious climate in unexpected ways. A couple of local Catholics from Neston, Tony and Gladys Moreton, began to style themselves as Teresa Higginson's 'worldwide promoters' and renewed the publishing of pamphlets, prayer-cards and leaflets in the 1980s. The Moretons also advertised such events as 'private' pilgrimages to be held 'in thanksgiving' for the Sacred Head; prayers to be said at Teresa Higginson's graveside; and books – most notably Ann Pitts and Sr Mary Dolores' *Teresa Helena Higginson: Servant of God* (Neston, 1986) – to be published to further the cause. They even arranged for her 'relics' to be put on display at St Alexander's Church in Bootle.

Margaret Rainford, writing from Ormskirk, Lancashire, in 2009, claimed Teresa Higginson's life to have been 'a testimony of fidelity and holiness'. Declaring her beatification to have been 'temporarily blocked, not rejected outright', she hinted that 'a striking miracle would certainly move things to be reconsidered' and help to revive her as 'an example for all teachers'.[111] Thanks

108 Edinburgh, Scottish Catholic Archives, DG/9/10/2: Unpublished letter from Archbishop of Liverpool to Edward Lonsdale, Teresa Higginson Association, 11 January 1945.

109 Ibid., DG/9/10/2: Unpublished letter from Archbishop of Liverpool to Edward Lonsdale, Teresa Higginson Association, 27 February 1945.

110 Ibid., ED 24/14/1: Unpublished letter from B. McVey (McClusky) to the Holy Father, 2 October 1951.

111 Margaret M. Rainford, Letter to the Editor, *Catholic Herald*, 19 June 2009, 13.

to the popular rise of the Internet in Britain from the 1990s, the Moretons' message was picked up by various blogs and websites, and new hagiographies, such as those published by Michael Hutchings in 2000 and Richard Whittington-Egan in 2010, continue to keep the 'cause' alive. Typing 'Teresa Higginson' into a search engine like Google currently (in 2014) calls forth some 271,000 references.

Conclusion

The public dispute over Teresa Higginson that emerged in the British Catholic community between the two world wars appears to have had many of the hallmarks of more celebrated clashes between self-conscious secularizers and traditional Christians that took place across the European continent. This time, however, the argument was, so to speak, kept within the Catholic family, largely turning over the question as to how far English Catholicism ought to admit the reductionist language of the newly emerging discipline of psychology into the realm of religious experience. The extent to which English Catholic professionals, including clergy, came to use medical language that was characteristic of anticlerical attacks in the Francophone world is striking. Rather than draw on discourses of rationality, empiricism and neurology to discredit the supernatural, however, English Catholics did so principally to protect the good name and reputation of their Church and their faith in what was perceived to be a predominantly Protestant and increasingly secular-minded world. Dr Walshe, like other influential English Catholic professionals, vowed to 'fight', for as long as necessary, for the cause of 'rational religion as against miraculism, for faith as against credulity'.[112]

The cause for the beatification of Teresa Higginson forced Catholics in Britain to think hard about the nature of their faith and to take sides in what were sometimes presented as two rival approaches to Catholic truth, one ostensibly more coolly intellectual and the other supposedly more emotional and credulous. Although often presented by historians as simple dichotomies based on social class, ethnicity or gender, modern English, Scottish and Irish Catholic attitudes towards the miraculous appear in practice to have been far more individual. The cause for the beatification of Teresa Higginson touched a Catholic nerve. The physical manifestations of mysticism that she presented to the Catholic world could be taken as either a 'sign' of supernatural favour or as a 'symptom' of neurological complaint. In England, self-consciously progressive Catholics succeeded in persuading the Vatican to declare her case inexpedient. But the divisions that her case exposed within the Catholic community in Britain proved to be resilient. Local Catholic support for the cause of

112 Walshe, Letter to the Editor, *The Tablet*, 26 February 1938, 278.

Teresa Higginson has not entirely disappeared, even today. Nor, more than a century after Teresa Higginson's death, has it adopted the 'rational' discourse favoured by those prominent English Catholic clerics and laypeople who managed to block the Cause in 1938. Not only do a small but energetic group of Liverpool and Lancashire Catholics continue to hope that the 'local saint' from the Wirral may one day be canonized and English Catholic teachers gain their special patron: they also accept the 'testimony' for diabolical wrangles, mystical union and stigmata far more readily than did Teresa Higginson's Victorian Catholic contemporaries.

DISENCHANTED AMERICA

ACCOUNTING FOR THE LACK OF EXTRAORDINARY MYSTICAL PHENOMENA IN CATHOLIC AMERICA

PAULA KANE

Scholarship in history often begins with a 'cultural predicament', as historian and ethnographer James Clifford claimed of his own work a quarter century ago.[1] As scholars identify certain predicaments – by which Clifford meant the study of identities experiencing rapid cultural change as they come in contact with different cultures – they re-evaluate their own assumptions, using such exercises to unearth new data and new interpretations of the relationship between the present and the past. Such exercises permit us to revision the past, not as a linear path to 'modernity', but as an uneven set of steps forward and back not inevitably destined to produce the present.

American Catholics represent an ethnoreligious group whose narrative would seem to be ideally suited to such an exercise. To this point, their history has relied heavily upon the model of cultural adaptation to modernizing forces within a national frame, resulting from the emigration of millions of European Catholics to the United States between 1845 and 1924. After 1965, new Catholic migrants arrived from Asia, Central and South America. It has been assumed that over several generations, these diverse immigrants were transformed from foreigners into ethnics and finally into Americans, their assimilation process reaching a critical tipping point at first in the 1920s and again in the 1960s as Catholics with European ancestors participated in ever increasing numbers in institutions that held economic, political and social authority. The latter stage of integration of American Catholics resulted from

1 See Clifford, *The Predicament of Culture*, but more useful here is his edited volume, *Writing Culture: The Poetics and Politics of Ethnography.*

several factors related to events that followed the Second World War, including the access of veterans to higher education guaranteed by the G.I. Bill, subsequent employment opportunities in white collar professions, and the construction of suburbs and new affordable housing which led urbanites out of their ethnic enclaves and into the new suburbs where they mixed with diverse ethnoreligious groups.

What the assumed assimilation of this emergent Catholic middle class has meant in terms of its religious identity in the modern era presents us with a cultural predicament worthy of Clifford's terms. For Catholics, has the process of 'becoming American' produced significant changes in the way that the European religious heritage of immigrants was understood and practiced? For this volume, I shall examine Catholics' relationship to a perceived modern American identity through their anti-modern belief in mystical phenomena in the nineteenth and twentieth centuries. Two questions follow: first, in order to integrate into a Protestant majority culture, did American Catholics abandon or alter some of their traditions and self-understanding? Second, did American Catholic instances of exceptional bodily mysticism help or hinder Catholic accommodation in the United States?

Mystical events with physical signs are usually considered to be a particular form of Catholic counter-modernity. Bodily experiences associated with Catholic mysticism (bleeding wounds, clairvoyance, ecstatic states, visionary revelations) have marked a robust difference from Protestant traditions since the Reformation era. As reports of miraculous events increased in the nineteenth century due to the Catholic Revival in Europe, they renewed theological and popular emphasis upon the unseen, the intuitive, the emotional, and the supernatural. The dramatic increase of reports of mystical phenomena in Europe was noticeably lacking in America, however. In Europe, such phenomena even experienced a new peak in the 1800s, seen in numerous Marian apparitions and reports of at least twenty stigmatics, a pattern that continued in the following century.[2] At the same time in the United States, by contrast, I have located only a few reports of mystical phenomena, mostly fraudulent. The first and only American Marian vision to receive Vatican approval, for instance, was an 1859 apparition to a Belgian nun in Wisconsin, which was only formally recognized in 2010, and which remains largely unremarked.[3] It is un-

2 Statistics on Marian apparitions compiled by the International Marian Research Institute (IMRI) at the University of Dayton chart a peak of Marian visions in the thirteenth century (772), but only 26 in the seventeenth century. A new Marian fervour that emerged in the nineteenth century, endured through the twentieth, characterized by a more diverse audience and few Vatican approvals. Data from The Mary Page of IMRI at <www.udayton.edu/imri>.

3 Sister Marie Adele Joseph Brise (1831-1896), via websites and information at the Green Bay Diocesan Archives. The shrine is called Our Lady of Good Help (www.ourladyofgoodhelp.com), located in Champion, Wisconsin, also called Robinsonville.

clear if any alleged American stigmatics (1891, 1922) were genuine. Although miraculous cures were the most commonly reported supernatural event, their verification was never institutionalized in America in the same way as at the Lourdes Medical Bureau.

Forgetting the past in order to fit in?

Following from the two questions raised above about the cultural role of mysticism for American Catholics, this chapter will examine the scarcity of extraordinary corporeal phenomena through several eras of Catholic identity-formation in the United States by asking if mystical experience was discouraged or diluted in America because it ran counter to assimilative goals. Second, using various types of mystical events – Marian apparitions, supernatural healing, stigmatization, Eucharistic miracles and exorcism – I shall ask if they represent a continuity or rupture with Old World traditions. Additionally, because mysticism and sainthood have an historical connection in Catholicism, it is significant that the handful of Americans who have been canonized, such as Frances Cabrini and Elizabeth Ann Seton, have not been chosen because of their mystical experiences, but as representatives of heroic virtue through their selfless service to others. This pattern would seem to indicate that by the late twentieth century, mystical encounters were indeed downplayed in the American church.

A recent set of essays on modern American Catholics has highlighted the middle decades of the twentieth century as marking the definitive moment of Catholic integration in the social, political and economic spheres of the United States. Catholic achievement of a high degree of assimilation also paralleled America's rise to dominance as the western superpower. *Catholics in the American Century: Recasting Narratives of U.S. History* suggests that Catholics became participants in the so-called 'American Century' by connecting their tradition of natural law theology and the natural law tradition of the nation's founders. This intellectual manoeuvre bolstered the Catholic citizens' sense of belonging and helped them resolve their 'concern with perennial principles and their suspicion of relativism'.[4] The volume's editors claim that 'how these Catholic ideas and institutions at once inhibited and facilitated assimilation to U.S. society is the central drama of twentieth-century U.S. Catholic history'.[5] In short, they take up Clifford's 'predicament' of rapid social change as Catholics experienced it intellectually during an era of reduced religious tensions and increased educational and economic opportunities.

4 McGreevy, 'Introduction', 2.
5 Ibid., 5.

The opening chapter of that collection highlights tensions and ambiguities between Catholics and their Protestant antagonists. Traditionally, the Protestant ethos of individualism and self-reliance has been at odds with Catholic principles of serving the common good and of loyalty to Rome. Given the European origins of most American Catholics, in his contribution to the volume Robert Orsi ponders how Catholics *are* Americans and asks whether 'the break between the ancient and the modern was as sharp as the changes from the Latin to the English Mass made it seem' after Vatican II.[6] While much of Orsi's essay studies a cultural factor – the uses of memory by pre-Vatican II Catholics – via the theories of French anthropologist and philosopher Bruno Latour, it suggests that because Catholics were challenged about their suitability as American citizens, they actively 'purified' their past and suppressed their Otherness in creating their own historical narratives to match or partner with dominant Protestant notions about the identity of the United States.[7] In short, a deliberate effort of forgetting the past seemingly accompanied the Catholic road to Americanization. In positive terms, other American historians propose that Catholics remained 'somewhat askew' to the dominant culture and to modernity in adopting an 'off-modern' identity.[8] These terms offer synonymous ways of describing the uneven passage of Catholics to modernity, even while 'modernity' cannot be the assumed core or goal of American identity.

Catholics' efforts at fitting in were only partly successful, however, as were their efforts to suppress cultural memory. In Orsi's revisionist narrative, New World Catholics continued to draw upon ancient Catholic traditions of spiritual strength, physical suffering and martyrdom to construct their version of American history, intended to reveal and support their patriotism. Catholic immigrants and their children strove to embrace the national ethos but also *challenged* it by use of these three themes. While Protestant Anglo-Saxons had assumed that their providential vision of America was secured by their split from the Roman Church in the seventeenth century, Catholic Americans responded over time by installing their own heroes into civic chronicles to highlight those who showed through their endurance of persecution, pain and sacrifice that *they* were the nation's true chosen people.[9] The result was that Catholics worked through a variety of strategies before finding ways to assert their patriotism while maintaining a distinct self-understanding. This interpretation implies that by the 1960s, American Catholics had achieved a delicate balance between insider and outsider identity.

A somewhat different inflection of the relationship between Protestants and Catholics comes from historian Jon Gjerde, whose posthumous work,

6 Orsi, 'U.S. Catholics between Memory and Modernity', 33.

7 Ibid., 14.

8 Orsi uses the term 'somewhat askew', while Stephen Schloesser has coined the phrase 'off-modern'. Schloesser, *Jazz Age Catholicism*, Prologue.

9 Orsi, 'U.S. Catholics between Memory and Modernity', 33.

Catholicism and the Shaping of Nineteenth-Century America (2012), argued that the best way to understand these two antagonists is to study how they were in conversation with each other. He contends that the arrival of Catholic immigrants from the 1840s onward forced Protestants to figure out how to integrate them, leading to the paradox that 'the growth of pluralism in the United States was fostered by efforts to create a homogeneous nation'.[10] In certain fields – the nature of family life and the role of women – there were areas of intersection and agreement between the two Christian traditions. In other realms, such as social and economic justice, Protestants and Catholics took starkly different approaches. But in all interactions, it was the constant encounter between the two traditions that profoundly shaped American modern society by setting the framework for analogous debates from the late nineteenth century to the present.[11]

I shall consider the implications of Clifford, Orsi and Gjerde for a chosen set of examples of Catholic mystical events reported in the United States between 1797 and 1937. This era precedes widespread Catholic assimilation that followed World War II, and instead encompasses the founding of the United States, when the Catholic population was negligible, to the early twentieth century, when Catholics comprised the largest single religion and more than 75% of the working class. Prior to mid-nineteenth century, there were fewer than twenty Catholic dioceses in the new United States and less than 400,000 Catholics. Yet one of the earliest spiritual dramas occurred on the Virginia frontier in 1797, near today's Martinsburg, West Virginia.[12] It combined elements of a haunted house, a dying stranger, a priest-exorcist, conversions, and enduring Reformation disputes.

The Wizard Clip

The episode began when a Lutheran family, headed by Adam Livingston, had migrated to a new site in Virginia after several farming failures in Pennsylvania. After Mr. Livingston denied a visiting stranger access to the last rites of the Catholic Church, the family home became haunted by evil spirits who cut and shredded their books, clothes, papers, and even leather boots and saddles. At the request of Livingston, Father Dennis Cahill came from Hagerstown, Maryland to say Mass twice at the house, which finally put an end to the household disturbances from the 'Wizard Clip', as the episode became known. Through the encouragement of a Catholic neighbour, Livingston converted to Catholi-

10 Gjerde, *Catholicism and the Shaping of Nineteenth-Century America*, 13.
11 Ibid., Editor's Epilogue, 257.
12 At the time, West Virginia was not yet a state, so the territory was part of Virginia. Details of these events come from Finotti, SJ, *The Mystery of the Wizard Clip*, and Laidley, 'Wizzard Clip'.

cism. Soon after, Prince (and priest) Demetrius Gallitzin (1770-1840), son of a German countess and a Russian royal ambassador, arrived in 'Cliptown' to investigate the reports of the supernatural shreddings. His presence initiated a distinctly un-American pattern of foreign-born aristocratic priests involving themselves in American mystical occurrences.

The second stage of the Livingston family drama unfolded with the sudden arrival of a mystical voice within their home that was audible to the household members. For the next seventeen years the family received religious instruction from the 'Voice', which educated them in Catholic doctrine, urged them to pray for the souls in Purgatory, and shrieked when experiencing the pangs of those already in torment in Purgatory. Other messages delivered by the Voice resembled Jansenist preachers of the seventeenth century, inveighing against women's taste for ostentation, but ultimately, the Voice led the Livingstons and others to become staunch Catholics, and even to proselytize neighbouring Catholics, Protestants and unbelievers. The Wizard Clip narrative is oddly de-centred, with the Livingston family representing one node; the neighbouring McSherrys another; Father Gallitzin and assorted Catholic bishops and priests yet another. The various stories were much later compiled by a Jesuit in the 1870s, and appeared in pamphlet form from Our Lady of the Rosary Library in Kentucky to fashion a coherent whole out of a bewildering series of events. The narrative minimized the poltergeist shreddings in preference for the conversion of Protestants. In 1904 the *West Virginia Historical Magazine* wrote about it, and during the Great Depression, the Works Progress Administration which produced guidebooks on the histories and notable events and places of each state, covered the Wizard Clip in its 1941 volume on West Virginia. As recently as 2008 'The Mystery of the Wizard Clip' pamphlet was republished by a conservative Catholic pamphleteer, with the addition of 'Questions and Answers on Salvation' written in 1875 by a traditionalist Redemptorist priest.

Catholics understood the peculiar episode of the Wizard Clip in multiple ways: as proof of God's existence; as evidence that Roman Catholicism was the only source of salvation; and as a call to spiritual revival for the tepid churchgoer. Latter-day commentators noted that the Voice successfully warmed the hearts of former Protestants and made many conversions on the Pennsylvania, Virginia, and Maryland frontier. These conversions may be regarded alongside the more than 10,000 converts credited to Father Gallitzin, the 'Apostle of the Alleghenies', who was himself a convert from the Orthodox Church or, more likely, from the strident rationalism of his father.[13]

The Wizard Clip conversions, which preceded the massive influx of European Catholics, do not fit Orsi's model for immigrant Catholics of the latter

13 Gallitzin's cause for canonization became active in 2005, when he was named a Servant of God. See 'Official Site: Canonization of Prince Demetrius Gallitzin', *The Cause for Canonization of Servant of God Demetrius Gallitzin*. 2005, <www.demetriusgallitzin.org>.

part of the century. The small band of Catholics of the newborn United States did not harp on the merits of suffering or martyrdom, traits that became more characteristic of the devotional piety of 1880 to 1950. They did, however, reflect Gjerde's model of two Christian traditions confronting each other, using individual conversions as their battleground, often in borderland areas where Protestants were alarmed about a Catholic takeover. The Voice's overriding theme was the truth of Catholic beliefs against rivals, and the need to save souls in Purgatory through prayer. Frontier Catholics were carving out a place for themselves in a Protestant land, converting others by example of their piety, with help from God's direct and miraculous intervention on their behalf, speaking through the Voice.[14] They answered the contempt of their Protestant rivals by claiming the conversions as triumphs over prejudice.[15]

Mary's first appearance in the United States

As the American frontier moved further west, a second nineteenth-century example of extraordinary mystical phenomena was the apparition of the Virgin Mary to a Belgian immigrant in the wilds of Wisconsin in October of 1859. Arrayed in 'dazzling white', Mary requested Adele Brise (1831-1896) to 'Gather the children in this wild country and teach them what they should know for salvation... Teach them their catechism, how to sign themselves with the sign of the Cross, and how to approach the sacraments...'[16] The Virgin's initial concern for proper observation of ritual practices showed little concern for the opinions of outsiders, focusing instead upon evangelization of sinners and instruction of the faithful, that they might not lose their religion in a new place. Brise set about establishing St Mary's Boarding School for children, and teaching there with fellow Franciscan tertiaries. But in her third appearance, Mary identified herself to Brise as 'the Queen of Heaven who prays for the conversion of sinners'. Since Brise's visions occurred one year after those of Bernadette Soubirous in Lourdes, France, it seems likely that they were an imitation by the Belgian immigrant, including an affirmation of a Marian title (Queen of

14 In the first American Catholic novel, *Father Rowland* (1829), by Jesuit Charles Constantine Pise, the plot is a thinly-disguised doctrinal defense of Catholic principles against Protestant critics and particularly a rebuttal to the anti-Catholic novel, *Father Clement* (1823).

15 The fear of Catholic conversion of the West inspired Calvinist minister Lyman Beecher (1775-1863) to write the tract, 'Plea for the West' (1834), which he delivered in sermon form numerous times and which led to the burning of the Ursuline Catholic convent in Boston in 1834.

16 From Bishop David Ricken's 'Decree on the Authenticity of the Apparitions of 1858 at the Shrine of Our Lady of Good Help', accessed online at <shrineofourladyofgoodhelp.com>. A scholarly interpretation, utilizing original documents from the Green Bay Diocesan Archives, is Park, 'The Negotiation of Authority'. Edward Looney furnishes many details in 'Called to Evangelize'.

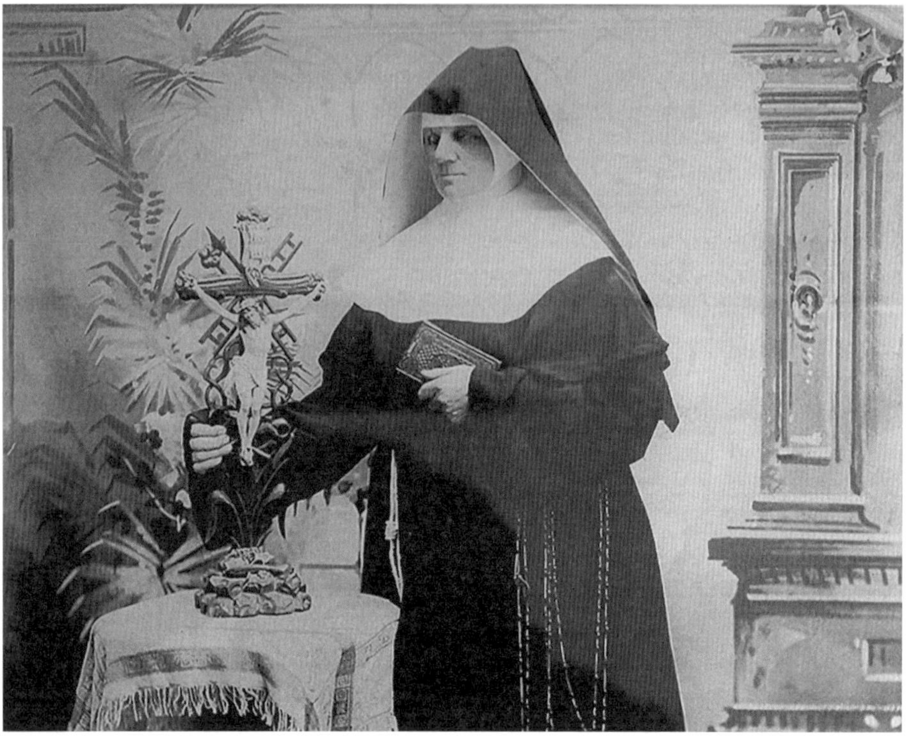

Adele Brise, c. 1870
[Champion (Wisconsin), National Shrine of Our Lady of Good Help]

Heaven versus Immaculate Conception), and the creation of a new pilgrimage chapel in America. Believers have drawn parallels between Brise's status as a poor woman and Bernadette's impoverished family, and the fact that Mary identified herself to each woman by a specific title. Bernadette entered a convent following her visions; Adele became a Third Order Franciscan, and so on. However, as Karen Park argues, evidence suggests that the La Salette visions of 1846 furnished the primary influence upon Brise. After Mary identified herself to Adele as the Queen of Heaven, she warned that Jesus' punishment of sinners was imminent, and remarked that 'I can hardly hold [back] his arm', echoing the Virgin's ominous warning at La Salette about the imminent destruction of the world.[17] This darker message about the consequences of human sinfulness was eliminated from the official apparition story put forward by the Diocese of Green Bay for the 2010 approval of the Brise apparition. Park shows how the bishop selectively eliminated details of Brise's narrative that did not fit the template of a pious, poor, woman who was always obedient

17 Park, 'The Negotiation of Authority', 9-12. Park points out that a broadside of the La Salette vision became widely available at the Lourdes shrine, and that the La Salette devotion was widely promoted by the nearby bishop of Grenoble, likely familiar to Brise in Brabant, Belgium, through the Catholic press. Ibid., 14.

to the priest. Because Brise refused to change her story of the grim message from Mary despite the threat of excommunication, which was eventually imposed upon her by the bishop. From the perspective of an emerging American Catholic Church, the several bishops' choice to edit out the harshness of the apparition represents a conscious choice to minimize mystical lore in favour of practical service to others.

As at the Wizard Clip, the Wisconsin visions had a second phase. Over time, the Shrine of Our Lady of Good Help flourished in Champion, Wisconsin at the apparition site. Pilgrims claimed miraculous healings and left a collection of crutches, as at Lourdes. A recent historical study suggests that Brise, the lone Marian visionary and shrine in the United States to receive Church approbation, was rendered uncontroversial through strategic shaping of her narrative by a series of bishops, so that she easily met with Church approval.

A new era of Catholic confidence

By the early twentieth century, American Catholics followed the lead of its episcopacy (from the decrees of the 1884 Plenary Council of Baltimore) in other more obvious pragmatic plans: to build a separate Catholic subculture whose institutions would envelop each Catholic from birth to death. This counter-assimilative strategy, focused upon constructing new parishes schools, colleges, convents, and hospitals, often presented Catholics as superior to other groups in the decades before they fully joined the 'American century' after World War II. A Catholic triumphalist mentality, which flourished because of these expansionist efforts, undergirded the reception and interpretation of a third example of embodied mysticism: the reported stigmatization of an Irish-American woman from New York City. At the same time, the investigation of Margaret Reilly (1884-1937) brought European debates between religion and scientific investigation into the American context and fashioned a local-global connection.

An American stigmatic

Reilly had tried several times to enter convent life in Manhattan, but had been turned away by several orders due to her poor health. She ultimately succeeded in joining the Congregation of the Good Shepherd at its convent in Peekskill, New York.[18] She experienced paralysis of her legs once she arrived there, and never walked again. She was possibly marked by the wounds of Christ

18 I study the case in *Sister Thorn and Catholic Mysticism in Modern America*. Details about Margaret Reilly/Sister Mary of the Crown of Thorns come from this source.

between 1922 and her death in 1937, making her the first American stigmatic.[19] Although Reilly's final vows were delayed by controversy over her mystical claims, she became Sister Mary of the Crown of Thorns in 1928, persevering in her vocation through chronic illness for the next decade until her death. She was regarded by some as a genuine mystic and by others as a self-serving fake. After her death her followers (numerous Irish among them) hoped to put her forward as the first American saint, but the cause never materialized beyond the local level. Nonetheless, the element that makes Sister Thorn suitable for this chapter is her presence as one of very few instances of corporeal mysticism in the United States. Her stigmata represent a far more physical experience than the locutions at the Wizard Clip or the apparitions in Wisconsin and, as it turned out, a greater transnational phenomenon.

Sister Thorn's stigmatization transcended nationalism because she was investigated by European commentators and some clergy who were themselves recent arrivals to America. The web of connections that resulted from their interaction forged a transatlantic community among priests, sisters, entire religious orders, physicians, and laity as they strove to match Sister Thorn's experiences with the template of preceding *stigmatisées*. Local news media clamoured for information, but without access to the convent, resorted to sensationalism. Notably, journalists compared Margaret with the few Europeans known already in the American press, such as the Tyrolean mystics Maria Domenica Lazzari and Maria Mörl; Anne Catherine Emmerich of Westphalia and Louise Lateau of Belgium.

As Adele Brise's visions had been redacted by bishops into a story about female submission, so the raw data about Sister Thorn's visions and wounds was even more quickly transformed into a narrative dominated by suffering. Sister Thorn's spiritual practices included plentiful examples of extreme self-mortification which merely served to highlight her sanctity for her contemporaries, while the unsettling details of her confrontations with demons were edited out. Her case reveals the themes of pain and martyrdom described in

19 In 1891 Mrs. Mary Stuckenborg of Louisville, Kentucky, a convert, claimed to receive the stigmata, and was observed at an infirmary by priests and later by local pastors and physicians. Her trance states attracted attention, as did the regularity of her stigmatizations every Friday for more than 100 weeks. *The Galveston Daily News* reported that 'efforts have twice been made to give the mysterious case a thorough scientific examination, but the plans could not be carried out, though they have not yet been abandoned' (15 March 1893, p. 5). Another paper said of Stuckenborg that 'for years she was an inmate in the lowest bawdy house in the city'. In addition to the Texas and Kentucky press, notices about Stuckenborg appeared in dailies as diverse as Clarksville, Tennessee; Staunton, Virginia; St. Paul, Minnesota; Wichita, Kansas; Sacramento, California; Abbeville, Louisiana; and Wheeling, West Virginia. Often, stories quoted some prior source nearly verbatim; very few provided verifiable details. The Louisville bishop, McCloskey, had visited Louise Lateau some years earlier, which may account for his insistence upon a thorough medical examination of Stuckenborg.

Orsi's discussion of the generation of Catholics of the 1920s-40s who were poised between immigrant and American identities, but her existence also reflected Gjerde's question about the perennial 'conundrum' facing American Catholics, namely 'how they could be pluralist and liberal, on the one hand, and particularistic, on the other'.[20] Sister Thorn's wounds and visions were moulded by the Church to support orthodox belief, by drawing connections to Christ's Passion and to support the Eucharistic piety and the cult of the Sacred Heart that flourished in popular devotions. Moreover, she represented the victim spirituality that was popular among Catholics during her lifetime, an individual's acceptance of extreme suffering to vicariously suffer on behalf of another or others. Sister Thorn's own painful death from pancreatic cancer was regarded as further proof of the marvels of suffering, marking a different emphasis given to her life than the events at the Wizard Clip a century earlier.

In the 1920s it was no accident that Sister Thorn's followers had one eye on her, and one on the nation's non-Catholics. From the 1880s Catholics had been engaged in building a parallel history of the U.S. by employing persecution, pain and sacrifice in order to reclaim national history for their own. These efforts did not mean that they were unconcerned about Protestant opinion. In light of recent speculations by historians about the contrast between Catholic memory and modernity, we may ask how Catholics explained the disparity between the two. If Catholics never quite acceded to an American history that was defined by Protestants, then did they fail to become modern as well, because they persisted in belief in apparitions, miracles, and stigmata? Orsi claims that because Catholics were 'impure citizens' who would never completely fit in, they relied on past motifs of martyrdom, pain, and suffering to guide what they valued as important.[21] The advocates of Sister Thorn found these ingredients in abundance in her life, and highlighted them for the public. They received further support from international events: the crisis of the Great War (1914-1918) had only added fuel to the Church's conviction that belief in the supernatural was a necessary rebuke to 'modernism'. Sister Thorn's devotees reacted to her in this way and circulated stories about her in support of this view.

Before considering other types of exceptional mysticism reported in America, Sister Thorn's existence in the United States prompts two further questions: why were few stigmatizations recorded in American history, given the central role of Christ's Passion in Catholic piety? And why did the 'objective' observation of her stigmata eschew the use of photography, psychology and scientific measures? Thorn's supporters included Catholics who energetically shared information between America and Europe via correspondence

20 Gjerde, *Catholicism and the Shaping of Nineteenth-Century America*, 67.

21 I would argue that Jews could claim even greater impurity since, unlike Catholics, they were not part of the Christian majority in America.

and scholarship. Their actions can be seen in two lights: as a setback for Catholic integration in America by exposing a potentially off-putting dimension of Catholicism to a Protestant public, or as positively contributing to a Catholic global-local, or 'glocal'. (The sociological term implies that neither side of the equation has priority.)[22] Unlike the one-way flow of ultramontanism from the Vatican outward, for 'glocal' Catholicism, the European tradition did not necessarily trump the American. The bond was instead expressed in a two-way flow of religious men and women, sacred objects, publications, and ritual practices. The transnational spread of devotion to Sister Thorn was aided by a revival of mysticism that followed the First World War, which led to searches for connections to Christian mystics of the past. Although we cannot accurately claim that a global culture existed in 1900, yet the impact of colonization by Catholic states and Catholic missionaries remained a significant force in joining Europe and the United States to different parts of the world through the universal claims of religion. The local dimension of the 'glocal' consisted in the details and cultural circumstances that made Sister Thorn, and each stigmatic, unique.

In each of the three examples discussed above, the American bishops played a determining role by holding the power of approval for investigations of miraculous claims and by controlling access of visitors to stigmatics and visionaries. The hierarchy could hinder scientific observers by claiming that the Church must first conclude its own investigation, a common strategy to delay and obstruct. This was not always the case, however. The bishop of Louisville had no problem with allowing doctors to investigate the alleged stigmata of Mrs Stuckenborg, perhaps because he had seen Louise Lateau and was aware that the investigations sponsored by the Belgian Academy of Medicine did not unseat Catholic belief in stigmata. Sister Thorn demonstrated the more typical case of a 'mystic' who was likely to prove inconvenient for American Catholics given the anti-Catholic tenor of the nation in the 1920s. Her cautious archbishop prohibited visitors, forbid her congregation from talking about her, and limited access to a few priests who had received his prior approval. Her devout, however, had already found ways to imagine how a bleeding nun could advance Catholic interests as the centre of national claims to moral superiority.

22 Robertson, 'Glocalization: Time-Space and Homogeneity-Heterogeneity'.

The role of print culture

The American colonial period and early Republic were dominated by an English-speaking Protestant cultural majority.[23] When nearly two million Roman Catholic immigrants arrived in the 1840s and 1850s to challenge that consensus, Protestants responded harshly to Catholic pleas for toleration and religious freedom, despite the enshrinement of those principles in the nation's Bill of Rights. During the era of gradual assimilation, 1880-1940, American Catholics reported only a few instances of unusual corporeal phenomena that were reminiscent of the saints and mystics of medieval or early modern European Catholicism. A survey of the major American Catholic periodicals of the late nineteenth and early twentieth centuries turns up very few native examples, aside from stories commemorating the martyrdoms of seventeenth-century New France, which included portions of New York state and Canada.

American Catholic 'memory' of the past was cultural by necessity, since there was no firsthand experience of stigmatics, village saints, or longstanding traditions of Christmas markets, holy wells or public processions for Holy Week. Print culture, therefore, played a major role in creating a Catholic American identity in the nineteenth century by conveying texts and images and targeting different groups of readers by age and gender. After about 1870 Catholic journals and newspapers contributed a profusion of materials that could be printed and reprinted throughout the country. Common examples of this extensive media include the frequent retelling of the lives of the saints, mystics, and visionaries. Such reporting allowed American Catholics to express ultramontane sympathies or to identify with a remembered past through their reporting of mystical phenomena occurring in Europe, notably the apparitions at Lourdes in 1858 and the stigmatization of Louise Lateau in 1868. The press, secular as well as religious, helped shape how American Catholics learned of mystical events. One way to interpret this journalism is as a means to mediate the experience of rapid change, by turning to European religious traditions for comfort.

Cultural memory also differed across ethnic groups. In certain ways, group feeling was created on the cultural frontier of the United States by the religious congregations, foreign-born clergy, and lay tertiaries whose practices became those of devout Europeans. Although she was an Irish-American, Margaret Reilly's visions and mystical conversations incorporated saints from medieval continental Europe, such as Colette and Gertrude, while her own *vita* as recorded by a visiting Swiss monk freely added details from the life of nineteenth-century German stigmatics as Anne Catherine Emmerich to her own. Sister Thorn received further information about saints and mystics

23 Hutchinson, *Religious Pluralism in America*. Prior to 1820, 95% of American settlers were Protestant.

through biographies and prayers suggested to her by her spiritual directors, fellow sisters, Catholic publications, and texts read aloud during meals in the convent refectory.

American Catholic print culture was not well developed before about 1870, and relied primarily upon reprinting news from and about Europe, notably concerning the lives of nineteenth-century stigmatics like Anne Catherine Emmerich and Louise Lateau. Here, as in Orsi's model, the Catholic press did emphasize the women's anguish. The *Pittsburgh Catholic*, for example, singled out Emmerich's sufferings as 'aggravated by repeated official examinations and violent attempts at a cure'.[24] When Louise Lateau was profiled, the American secular and Catholic press quoted long passages from eyewitnesses to conveying her gentle melancholy and patient resignation while being poked and prodded by scientific experimenters.[25]

If the American hierarchy proved hesitant about how to present Sister Thorn to the public, the activity of foreign-born clergy in promoting her continued a pattern from the early nineteenth century and contributed to the glocalization or internationalization of Catholic mystical phenomena, even if the United States did not appear to be fertile ground for mysticism.[26] The issue of American Catholic contribution to global Catholicism was intensified in the early twentieth century, when the potential canonization of colonial era Catholics became an issue among competing factions anxious to establish their relationship with Vatican saint-makers.[27] Sister Thorn's story became globalized by importing certain dimensions of European stigmatic cults and then vernacularizing them. For example, Margaret received revelations from the Lord that addressed macro- and micro-conflicts. In one instance when Jesus told her that 'America is the grave of religious life', he touched the national anxiety among Catholic leaders about loss of vocations in the United States. When Jesus warned Margaret that it was shameful when sisters went outside the convent without permission, he addressed a local concern in New York and New Jersey about the abuse of rules in defiance of the 1917 Canon Law revisions which had increased strictness of cloister for women.

Using a hagiographic template for stigmatized women that was already well-established, combined with the category known as the 'victim soul' which was elaborated in the nineteenth century, twentieth-century Sister

24 'Anne Catherine Emmerich', *Pittsburgh Catholic*, September, 1874.

25 For example, 'Is it a miracle?', *Cleveland Daily Herald*, 6 November 1874, and 'Louise Lateau', *Pittsburgh Catholic*, 3 April 1869.

26 Cohen, 'Re-Viewing the Twentieth Century', 51. Other than immigration and nationalism, it does not directly engage the other large-scale processes set in motion by 1492. According to another contributor to *Catholics in the American Century,* those topics include 'exploration, settlement, enslavement, industrialization, immigration, nationalism, imperialism, environmental degradation'.

27 See Cummings, 'American Saints'.

Thorn's advocates hoped to add one of their own to the roster of saints.[28] The reception of Sister Thorn reveals how extraordinary corporeal phenomena were perceived and interpreted by some twentieth-century Catholics. In addition to her alleged stigmata, American history contains reports of other extraordinary bodily events, namely miraculous cures, visions and exorcisms. A brief survey of some of this material suggests how such events exemplified the local (vernacular), but also contributed to the production of a global Catholic identity.

Healing the sick

Far more common than stigmata in the United States were reports of healing miracles. Some 27 years after the Wizard Clip incident began, Catholics learned of seventeen long-distance cures by Prince Alexander von Hohenlohe of mostly convented women in Kentucky, Maryland and Washington, D.C. between 1824 and 1838. Hohenlohe (1794-1849), a priest and an aristocrat, already possessed a legacy of successful exorcisms and spiritual healings in his native Germany, and in France and the Netherlands. The prince was handsome, charismatic, and a target of British cartoonists who used him to continue a robust Reformation tradition of priest-bashing. From Germany Prince Hohenlohe cured Ann Mattingly, the sister of the mayor of Washington, who had suffered with cancer for seven years. She lived on in good health for the next 31 years. Mattingly's cure continued the Wizard Clip's model of extraordinary phenomena being effected by European agents (often priest-aristocrats). Catholics held out the Hohenlohe cures as proof that God's power could defy space and time, through the power of the consecrated host, the Real Presence of Christ. (Mattingly's cure occurred while ingesting communion at the request of Father Hohenlohe, at the very moment that he was saying Mass in Europe.)[29] Their mutual communion connected Europe and America in a most sacred way through the central ritual of the Catholic faith and scored points against Protestant's denial of transubstantiation, which can only occur through the instrument of the priest.

The ability (and even necessity) of immigrant priests to act as conduits of European traditions was heightened by the scarcity of both Catholics and priests in the early United States. The latter received sympathy among Americans for the push factors that had driven clergy from Europe following the po-

28 I borrow the concept of vernacularization from sociologist Peggy Levitt who mentions three types, of which I found the last one relevant here, namely taking core concepts, articulating them in locally appropriate ways and modelling new ways to put them into practice. Levitt, 'Religion on the Move', 171.

29 The events are chronicled in Schultz, *Mrs. Mattingly's Miracle*. One of the first treatments of the topic of the Hohenlohe cures is Curran, 'The finger of God is Here'.

litical revolutions of 1789, 1830, 1848 and 1870. An 1880 history of the diocese of Pittsburgh summarized those early decades: 'There was no little moving of priests from place to place in the early days of Catholicity among us, without any apparent reason or authority in many instances... not a few of these came to America owing to the disturbances in most of the countries of western Europe at the close of the eighteenth and the early part of the nineteenth centuries...'[30] Such clergy were not always certain who was their superior, and where they might do the most good, so they sometimes followed their own itineraries and motives, improvising and inventing.

The cure of Ann Mattingly and subsequently, of numerous Visitation nuns at their convent in Washington, D.C. engaged theological and cultural issues that represented the central conflicts between Protestants and Catholics. For the few existing American bishops, it raised a question addressed by many nineteenth-century Christian theologians: can miracles occur in the post-apostolic age or were they unique to the lifetime of Jesus Christ?[31] A second issue that was also mirrored in vernacular piety was the uniquely Catholic belief in the Real Presence of Christ in the Eucharist. One of the social uses of Ann Mattingly among Catholics hinted at popular desire for greater attention to both issues. Because Ann was a laywoman, she could more readily serve as a public symbol of the truth of Catholic Eucharistic doctrine at a moment and in a place – the nation's capital – where Catholics were anxious to achieve public recognition and approval. As Nancy Schultz found in her study of the Mattingly healing, since the foreigners involved were 'enthusiasts', while the native Maryland Catholics tended to be moderates, it fell to Irish-born John England, who became bishop of Charleston, South Carolina, to chart a path that would satisfy both camps, using 'a rational and evidence-based examination' of the Mattingly cure.[32] Mattingly's case, therefore, became the earliest attempt to document miraculous healing in the United States.

The priest-physician

The healing ministry of a Belgian priest-physician that began in Pennsylvania in the 1870s presents a third occasion when American Catholics credited miraculous healings to a foreign-born priest. Like Fathers Gallitzin and von Hohenlohe, Suitbert Mollinger (1828/30-1892) of Mechelen, Belgium, had elite credentials. His Dutch Protestant father had served the King of Holland as prime minister, and had provided his son with an excellent 'liberal education'. After medical training in Naples, Rome and Genoa, Mollinger entered the Cath-

30 Lambing, *A history of the Catholic Church.*
31 Schultz, *Mrs. Mattingly's Miracle.*
32 Ibid., 153.

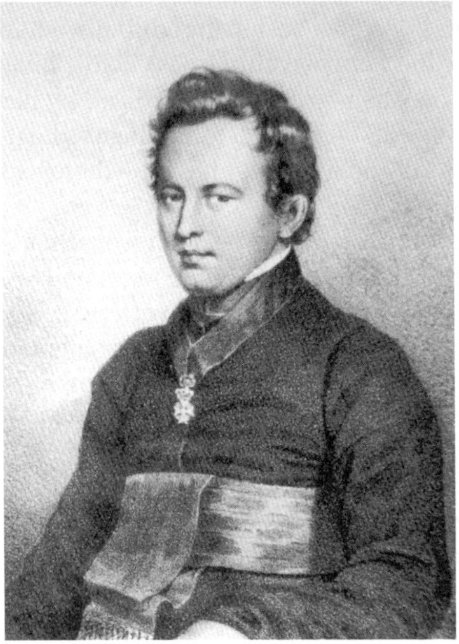

Prince von Hohenlohe. Lithograph by J. S. Decker.
[*Vienna, Österreichishe Nationalbibliothek*]

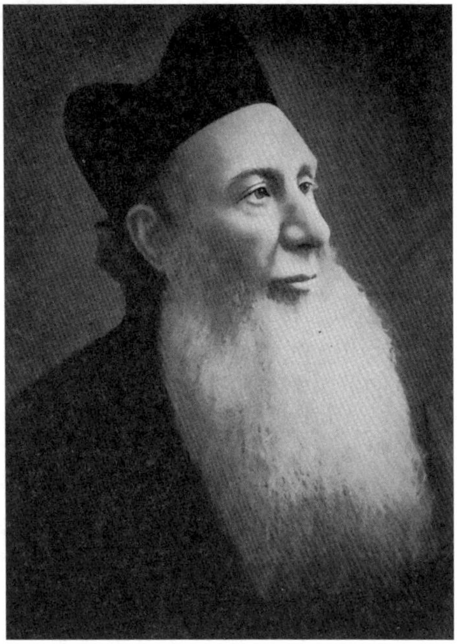

Father Mollinger.
[*USGenweb Archives*]

olic seminary in Ghent, which estranged him from his family. There he met an American bishop who sought volunteers for missionary work in America. Mollinger came to the United States in 1854, leaving New York City for Latrobe, Pennsylvania in 1857, where he was ordained for the diocese of Pittsburgh in about 1859. In 1868 he became pastor of Most Holy Name of Jesus church in the Troy Hill neighbourhood of the city. There he began to hold healing services whose popularity only increased over the next two decades. In 1890, the *New York Times* reported, at least 10,000 people convened at Mollinger's church on 13 June, the feast of St Anthony of Padua, to be healed. (That day was chosen because a relic of the saint is housed at the church and because Anthony was Mollinger's patron saint.) The rectory and the new St Anthony Chapel at the parish had been funded by Mollinger from an inheritance from his uncle and completed two years earlier to house the considerable collection of relics that the priest had purchased in Europe to rescue them from destruction by Bismark's *Kulturkampf*. The more than 7,000 relics assembled by Mollinger are described as the largest such collection in North America. At the priest's annual healing ceremonies, a 'curious assemblage of the lame, deaf, and blind' travelled from as far away as British Columbia, Canada to wait in the heat for their chance to be cured. Over time, ill persons and their families rented rooms in boarding houses in the neighbourhood for the mere chance to be near the priest. From Kansas came a typical report of a 'sad scene' for a blind woman who 'wanted to go to Father Mollinger, the Pennsylvania priest who claims to heal by supernatural powers', but who was regrettably 'convinced by her friends that it would be useless'.[33] Near the end of his career, Mollinger's healings also attracted many Americans from Kentucky and Tennessee, where had performed successful cures in years past.

Father Mollinger, who held medical credentials, devised a novel scheme for success in America: inside his parish church, he celebrated Mass and led the healing rites on certain days; outside, he directed patients (with prescriptions written in cypher) to the adjacent pharmacy which sold his own patented herbal medicines. By his own account, people were healed not because of him, but by seeing the relics, experiencing the laying on of hands, and the power of God. Following Mollinger's death in 1892, the sale of medicines was supposed to cease, following the bishop's directive. However, two pharmacists eventually competed for the clients at the Pittsburgh chapel, and sued each other in 1892 over control of medicinal compounds. The pharmacy continued to operate. Because no will was found for Father Mollinger, several family members arrived from Europe and stripped the chapel and rectory of all portable valuables, while the contest over the priest's pharmaceutical legacy continued. More than thirty years after the pastor's death, a Mollinger Medicine Company was incorporated in Pennsylvania in 1925, indicating that the business survived nonetheless. Advertisements for Mollinger's herbal pills and tinctures can be found in the Pittsburgh press in the 1920s, promising relief from catarrh, gout, lumbago, rheumatism and nearly every human affliction.

The combination of priest-doctor is unusual in America, and according to a Pittsburgh cleric, there were 'only one or two priest-physicians' in the country during Mollinger's heyday.[34] Yet Mollinger was a familiar type in Europe, especially in Bavaria. While Father Mollinger confounds our sense of an expert weighing in on the side of 'sign' or 'symptom' because he engaged both, his use of herbal medicines continued a robust European tradition of natural plant and water-based methods of healing. The best-known priest-naturopath, also from southern Germany, was Sebastian Kneipp (1821-97), whose mineral bath salts, skin lotions, whole grain bread and herbal teas are still available. Kneipp, who was ordained at age 30, became one of the founders of the naturopathic movement, and used hydrotherapy to help his poor country parishioners, after his own cure from tuberculosis as a young man. He later incorporated dietary and exercise elements into his regime to create an early form of naturopathy. By 2010 his popular book, *My Water Cure* (1886/1890), had achieved 74 editions in 10 languages. Pope Leo XIII was among his clients.

33 'There was a sad scene in Dr. Campbell's office yesterday', *The Atchinson Daily Globe*, 1 August 1891.

34 'The Dead Priest', *The Pittsburg Press*, 16 June 1892.

Kneipp dispatched his student, Benedict Lust (1872-1945) from Baden at the turn of the century, to introduce naturopathy in the United States, coinciding with the apex of Mollinger's ministry in Pennsylvania. *The Pennsylvania Medical Journal* praised 'men like Mollinger and Kneipp', who successfully cured patients after the physician had failed.[35] This example of Catholic glocalism contributes to the pattern by which American Catholics proved to be fertile ground for imported practices.

Divine healing has been claimed by many Christian traditions, but exorcism is a ritual associated uniquely with Catholic tradition and the priest's power to expel demons. It often produced violent results, as devils departed from the body of the possessed person. A well-documented case in Ealing, Iowa in 1928 involved Father Theophilus Riesinger (1868-1941), a Bavarian-born Capuchin who claimed to eject thousands of demons from the body of 40-year old Emma Schmidt. The events served in part as inspiration for William Blatty's famous novel that became the film, *The Exorcist* (1973). Much of the documentation of the Iowa exorcism came not from physicians, but from eyewitnesses in the community and the sisters at the Franciscan convent where the rites took place over a series of months. Several pamphlets were printed in Germany afterwards, and then translated into English six years later by a Benedictine monk in Minnesota. The pamphlets became widely distributed by sale to Catholic and secular audiences. The exorcism did not produce a national outcry against Catholic credulity in belief in devils or possession, however. Instead, Protestant and Catholic commentators alike remarked upon the exorcism as genuine proof of the existence of Satan. Some of the exorcist's predictions for the future identified the anti-Christ as arising in the 1950s, an apocalyptic theme that was later echoed by Cold War Marian visionaries and Protestant fundamentalists.

As related above, European clergy (here, represented by Belgian, Bavarian, and German-Russian priests rather than the more plentiful Irish) had a notable impact as agents and mediators of extraordinary phenomena in America. Yet the contemporary era has been marked by a shift away from clergy-centred events, as illustrated by the explosion of lay visionaries since the 1950s. Between 1949 and 1993 there were more than 30 reports of Marian visions in America, including Nancy Fowler (Conyers, Georgia); Mary Ann van Hoof (Necedah, Wisconsin); Veronica Lueken (Bayside, New York); Estela and Reyes Ruiz (Phoenix, Arizona); and Gianna Talone (Scottsdale, Arizona and Emmitsburg, Maryland). Talone, to take one example, was prohibited from continuing her activities in the Archdiocese of Baltimore after investigations found nothing of supernatural origin in her experiences.[36] In an instance of

35 Mayer, 'Hysteria in Children', *Pennsylvania Medical Journal*, 2 (1899) 9, 480-481.

36 The document appears at <http://www.archbalt.org/news-events/press-releases/alleged-apparitions.cfm>.

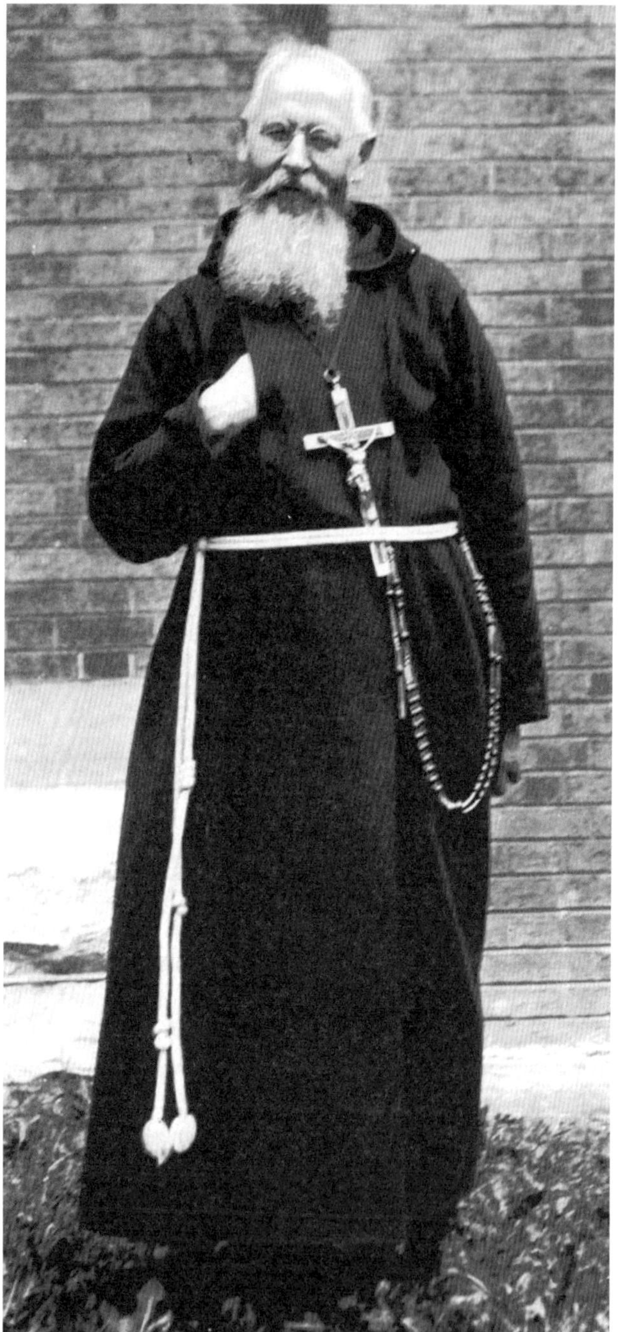

The Iowa exorcist, Father Riesinger
[*New York, Province of St Mary of the Capuchin Order*]

glocalism, Talone's initial visions were inspired by her visit to Medjugorje, a shrine in the former Yugoslavia that remains controversial, but that has strongly influenced American Marianism. The Marian apparitions during the Cold War and into the 21st century have placed individual seers at the centre of numerous spontaneous, but unapproved cults throughout the nation. Because American visionaries have often cited extra-American influences to strengthen their mystical claims, and have learned to master social media to communicate their messages, the Catholic hierarchy has had a hard time dispelling them.[37]

American exceptionalism?

Finally, was there something distinctively 'American' in the Catholic responses to extraordinary mystical phenomena, as described in the brief overview above? As discussed, some responses among American Catholics were closely shaped by unconventional immigrant, itinerant priests, whose impact included the introduction of relic cults, host miracles, devotion to the Miraculous Medal and Sacred Heart of Jesus, exorcisms, and hydropathy. American bishops, who were expected to be wary about the opinion of Protestants, were not necessarily at odds with the newly-arriving European-born priests on these matters since some, like Mollinger, performed the useful work serving German-speaking Catholics in Pennsylvania where monolingual priests could not. The immigrant or visiting priests were often the carriers of 'lived' or 'vernacular' piety from their homelands, rather than defenders of a strictly rational orthodoxy. The distinction between 'American' and foreign-born Catholics seemed not to matter in the investigation of mystical events. When the foreign-born Adele Brise experienced a vision of the Virgin in the United States, she closely imitated the La Salette apparition, followed by Lourdes-style healings at the emergent shrine.

There is an additional set of issues that derive from cultural questions about extraordinary events in the American Church. In the ongoing scholarly debate about the nature of American Catholicism (was it unique or derivative?), American Catholics contributed to the global identity of their tradition in the nineteenth and twentieth centuries through their attempts to establish a record of supernatural events, while at the same time, the social environment of Protestant individualism also weighed as a factor in how Catholics tried to mould their representation for the American public. If Catholics did embrace the notion of the founding of America as a divinely-sanctioned project that qualified its citizens to lead the rest of the world, were mystical events limited in scope and number by local factors, or did Americans try to associate them-

37 Apolito, *The Internet and the Madonna.*

selves with a Eurocentric Catholic identity by embracing extraordinary phenomena, even if in small numbers? On the other hand, if American Catholics sought their audience among their fellow Catholics in Europe, were they trying to identify themselves as deserving members of an international religious community?

As we examine the twentieth century, the stigmatization of Margaret Reilly and other mystical phenomena in the United States illustrated the ambivalence of Roman Catholics about their modern milieu. Mystics provided constant irritation to Protestants by supporting a vision of America grounded in Catholic (irrational) values of physical courage, stamina and suffering. These values, which Orsi describes as representing a 'radically different ontology' among Catholics, explain the unique appeal of the lives of the saints and martyrs for American Catholics, and the fascination with pursuing life as a 'victim soul' for a young woman like Margaret Reilly.[38] Cultural memory offered Catholics many hagiographies, but with Adele Brise and Sister Thorn, Americans gained persons with extraordinary spiritual gifts from their own country.

Margaret Reilly's devotees combined civic and sacred expectations about sainthood. Her advocates in the 1930s and 1940s were excited to propose her as the first American saint, or as the first Irish-American saint. Their hopes were not out of line with other existing attempts to promote American saints who had far weaker claims to be American: the Mohawk Kateri Tekakwitha who died in 1680, and Elizabeth Seton, an Anglican convert in colonial Maryland, were put forward in the 1880s (the Seton cause began officially in 1907), but the first canonization of an 'American' did not occur until 1946: Frances Cabrini, an Italian immigrant, was honoured for her contributions to society that were charitable and practical rather than mystical. As historian Kathleen Cummings has found, that while it may seem 'counterintuitive that Catholics would choose to mediate their Americanness through saintly devotion, the very religious practice that appeared most alien to Protestant observers, there is no question that hagiography took on a decidedly American dimension in the early twentieth century as U.S. Catholics repackaged European saints for a U.S. audience and petitioned for the canonization of one of their own.'[39] North Americans grumbled about the Vatican's partiality to making saints in Central and South America, whose total stood at 17 by 1900. The beginnings of hemispheric competition added to the globalization of the Catholic faith in the twentieth century.

When Americans assert that the United States has a special mission, the claim usually rallies conservatives through an idealist notion that its divine purpose is to promote liberty or liberal democracy throughout the world. An examination of Catholic identity in the U.S. helps us to rethink an historio-

38 Orsi, 'U.S. Catholics between Memory and Modernity', 22.

39 Cummings, 'American Saints', 204.

graphical and interpretive issue: what is Catholic identity, especially in relation to the historical cultural dominance of Protestantism? After centuries of being Protestantism's Other, did Catholics eventually become Americanized by adopting the 'rational' and 'pragmatic' aspects of national identity demonstrably undergirded by Protestantism? Such a result would presume that the mystical elements of faith would be downplayed or relatively minimized. This examination of mystical events attributed to American Catholics has shown that a mixture of both strategies existed: Catholic leaders suppressed publicity about some such events as superstitious relics of the Old World, while popular piety often found ways to use them to mediate relationships with Protestants.[40]

Given the rich heritage of European miracles since the Middle Ages, one might expect parallel attempts to create such traditions in the United States. But in fact the American catalogue of extraordinary phenomena is extremely limited as compared with the continent. I have suggested that four factors accounted for this limitation. First, the bulk of European Catholics did not arrive until after 1850, with the peak years of immigration between 1880 and 1924, so smaller populations of Catholics did not provide enough robust audiences for mystical events. Next, the circulation of priests between Europe and the U.S. shaped American pious beliefs and practices beginning in the early nineteenth century by mediating and popularizing an otherwise short list of wonders. Third, from the Vatican's perspective, if the United States signified a Christian frontier not released from 'mission' status until 1907, it is hardly surprising that America would try to connect its few mystics to the Old World. Extraordinary corporeal mystical events produced in the United States no such clear-cut and polarized rationalist vs. revelationist camps as had emerged in Europe, most particularly in nineteenth-century France where secular scientists and neurologists fought against the Catholic Church. Yet there were some similarities: Protestant political and scientific elites regarded Catholics as superstitious and anti-scientific, whereas Catholic professionals often strove to be received into the Protestant establishment by not pandering to behaviours which male Church leaders often regarded both as hysterical and as threats to patriarchal authority. Hence, Catholic professionals adopted the very norms provided to them by Protestant rationalist culture. For example, the prominent Catholic physician who examined Sister Thorn, had received European medical training, and dutifully echoed his instructor's theories of female hysteria or neurasthenia.

The study of alleged corporeal phenomena was at once principled and insufficient in the United States. The arenas of conflict and discursive problems were established by debates between medical authorities, Catholic clergy and hierarchy and the lived experience of ordinary Catholics. It seems clear

40 Ibid., 231.

that American Catholics' reception of so-called miracles was different than in Europe, but it remains to be seen how Americans understood the porous relationship between mystic and patient; private and public modes of religious expression; emergent medical and psychological disciplines; and religious and national identity. Mystical phenomena were difficult to distil into patriotic symbols, but perhaps harder still to preserve as miracles.

THE MAD SAINT AS HEALER

THE ISLAMIC MAJNUN IN AL-KATTANI'S *SALWAT AL-ANFAS* AND IN FRENCH COLONIAL MEDICINE AND SOCIOLOGY

ELLEN J. AMSTER

The *majnun*, the mad saint of Islam, also called the *majdhub* (the attracted one) or the *bahlul* (the holy fool), is 'one possessed by *jinn*', the beings who exist parallel to mankind on earth in the Qur'an (72:1-28) and whom God 'created of the fire of a scorching wind' (15:28). In 1999, I interviewed a 95 year-old lady in the old city of Fez, who described her father as *majnun*. She explained that her father's intimacy with God opened his body to believing Muslim *jnun* (plural of *jinn*), which rendered him a source of God's blessing (*baraka*) in the material world:

> For seven years, he ate bread, and he ate *jawi* [an herb used as incense] and he drank tea with safran... The people who are in him (*an-nas li fihi*), those things, that is what they wanted, the believers that were in him, that's what they ate... Those [*jnun*] that are from God. [He was one of] the people of rotation (*an-nouba*). And whomever the turn comes to, and he who has the key, he opens the door.[1]

God's blessing, or *baraka*, unlocked the separation between this world and the divine. He could predict the future and tell passer-by their most intimate thoughts, in a surprising manner:

> That is just like some part of the newspaper from God... And when he finds a woman, he says, 'Hey man! Man! Show your face!' He says

1 Interview with the author, My K., 22 March 1999, Fez, Morocco.

> this to the woman. To the man he says, 'Woman, cover your face! Be ashamed!'... He had *baraka* in him... For example, you came, and he knew you. What was in your mind, he will tell you.[2]

He prayed in the city mosques, and the people came to touch him for relief from illness. 'When they opened the door of Mawlay Idris [mosque], you find the slaves of God... So the people came, they followed him, and they grabbed at him.' One night he invited the neighbours to his home for his own funeral, performed his ablutions, prepared his shroud, and sent for his daughter and her baby son:

> At ten o'clock at night, he invited them, and the Lord of Faith took His faith [he died]. They let the word be spread... That night they [washed his body] in rosewater and orange flower water, they made a new *ghasil* [platform for washing the dead] for him... And the guardians and the police, they told people, [don't grab him like that], you all want to tear him apart. And when they covered him again with a *qiswa* [burial cloth], they were pushing with their shoulders, and then they pulled off his clothes until he was left with only the shroud. And the slaves of God were out of their minds. Just the youths were holding him up, from hand to hand.

This mad saint is one example of the Islamic saint (*wali*), whose knowledge of God manifests as exceptional corporeal phenomena – flying, predicting the future, healing, and to evildoers, punishment by sudden pain, illness, blindness, and vomiting. The *wali* is the 'Friend of God', also called *murabit*: he who connects/binds, (in French, 'marabout'). The translation of *wali* as 'Islamic saint' originates with French visitors to North Africa who observed Muslim pilgrims visiting *awliya* (pl. of *wali*) for healing from a variety of physical, mental, and social afflictions – touching their bodies, swallowing their saliva, praying and sleeping in their tombs, and performing healing at the shrines. For French observers, Islamic shrine visitation (*ziyara*) resembled the Catholic cult of the saints, especially the pilgrimage to the Virgin's shrine at Lourdes. As this 1999 interview suggests, the people of Fez witnessed such miraculous healing well into the twentieth century.

A modernist, positivist, and French interpretation of the Islamic saint in general and the *majnun* in particular began with French physicians and *sociologues* sent on scientific mission to North Africa in the late nineteenth century. For French doctors, the *majnun* was mentally ill or a charlatan and his 'miracles' were a public hallucination. To Durkheimian *sociologues*, the *majnun* (and the *wali* generally) was an *homme-fétiche*, a fetish-man, a totem venerated by a society too primitive for rational knowledge of disease, the body,

2 Interview with the author, Mawlay A., 22 March 1999, Fez, Morocco.

or medicine. For the French colonizer, popular veneration of the *majnun* was irrefutable evidence of intellectual darkness. The fact that Moroccans would look to the mentally afflicted for healing demonstrated the absence of any science or medicine in Morocco, the irrationality of the Islamic religion, and the necessity for a positivist French civilizing mission.

Moroccan nationalists of the 1930s rejected French cultural chauvinism and colonial domination but repeated French positivist views of the *majnun*, for they adopted *salafiyya*, or Islamic modernism, from the East (*mashriq*). *Salafiyya*, a reformist philosophy of the late nineteenth century, used a positivist, Comtean theory of knowledge to define modernity, an epistemological shift that led to an Islamic hostility to Islamic mysticism, Sufism, and esoteric religious knowledge in general.[3] For Moroccan Muslim nationalists, the spectacle of the *majnun* was an anti-modern embarrassment, the emblem of a popular backwardness that prevented Morocco from achieving its modernity and a rightful place among the independent nations.

The majnun as healer, in Islamic hagiography and Moroccan medical narratives

With his bizarre speech, antinomian behaviour, and shocking appearance, the *majnun* has been an enigma to Galenic Islamic physicians of the medieval period, to French doctors of the protectorate period (1912-1956), and to contemporary anthropologists. Variously understood as a madman suffering an organic illness (Michael Dols), by contemporary anthropologists as one possessed by demons (Vincent Crapanzano), and by scholars of religion as a radical ascetic (Ahmet Karamustafa), the *majnun* has been treated as a mental patient, a fraud, and a penitent, but never as a healer.

In this chapter, we consider the *majnun* as a healer, and indeed, as a public healer, one who brings healing simultaneously to human bodies and to society.[4] Saints heal through knowing (*ma'rifa*), by seeing the human body as the isthmus between 'the oceans of God and the cosmos'. To understand such phenomena in depth, we turn to a three-volume hagiographical compendium by the Moroccan scholar Muhammad ibn Ja'far al-Kattani, a historical aggregate of centuries of textual and oral memory about the saints of the city of Fez, published in 1898, *Salwat al-anfas wa muhadathat al-akyas bi man uqbira min al-'ulama' wa al-sulaha' bi Fas* (Entertainment of the Souls and Discourse of the Sagacious Concerning the Scholars and Righteous Persons Buried in Fez).

3 For a discussion, see Amster, *Medicine and the Saints*, 7-8, 46. However, positivism is not *necessarily* incompatible with Sufism; see the works of 'Ali Sharia'ti (Rahnema, *An Islamic Utopian*) and Muhammad ibn 'Abd al-Kabir al-Kattani (Bazzaz, *Forgotten Saints*).

4 We borrow this concept from Africanist historian Steven Feierman, 'Healing as Social Criticism'.

Combining the *Salwa* of al-Kattani, oral interviews conducted with elderly residents of the city of Fez in 1998-2000, and the theological phenomenology of Islam, we recover the *majnun* as healer. As I have argued elsewhere, saint 'healing' was actually the saint's restoration of God's law (*shari'a*) to individuals and to society, a way of actualizing the human body as the isthmus (*barzakh*) between the divine and material worlds.[5]

In the *Salwa*, the city of Fez is protected by her saints from tyranny; the saints cause rain to fall and plants to spring from the earth. Without their knowledge, 'afflictions would flow forth onto the people of the earth like an inundation'[6] and the people would be 'blind like beasts'.[7] A small minority of these saints are *majnun*, and a typical biography of such a mad saint is Sidi Bu 'Iyad al-Waryaghli, who died in 1748 A.D.:

> *#82 Sidi Bu 'Iyad al-Waryaghli d. 1162 hijri,* (1748 A.D.)
>
> And among them [the awliya]: the aged *majdhub shaykh*, the lover, absent one, driven mad with love, the righteous *wali* through whom one receives *baraka*; Sidi Abu 'Iyad al-Waryaghli. He was called 'Ibn Khaldun' and was born, grew up, and lived in Fez.
>
> He was, may God accept him, in the beginning of his life very sharp-witted, a merchant who did business in the Qisariyya and elsewhere, and he loved strumming and playing the oud. He had family and relatives from Sudan. Then he came in communication with Shaykh Sidi al-Haj al-Khayyat the excellent [a Sufi scholar], buried in Al-Sharshur, and he served him three or four years, until Sidi al-Haj al-Khayyat died, and that shone upon him which shone [i.e. al-Waryaghli achieved Sufi knowledge, or *ma'rifa*].
>
> And he stayed always in the Sufi lodge where his *shaykh* was buried, and frequently visited the people of Wazzan [a famous Sufi order] and those related to them, until his condition became great [i.e. he became illuminated with advanced spiritual state]. A great trance fell upon him, and he did not differentiate between heat and cold, or between giving and withholding; he let fall all obligation, and did things which are frowned upon in *shari'a* like smoking and this kind of thing. He defecated on his clothes and on his legs, and entered the mosque and the Idrissid shrine like that, and he struck his feet against the furniture of the mosque and a spray of faeces would fly from him onto it, because his *jallaba* was very full of faeces. And every time you see him, he is masturbating himself with his left hand, whether in the mosque or in the street, standing or sitting.

5 Amster, *Medicine and the Saints*, Chapter 1.
6 Al-Kattani, *Salwat al-Anfas*, 38.
7 Ibid, 27.

> The people complained about him to the *qadi* [judge] of the time, Sidi 'Ali Bu 'Inan, who imprisoned him in the *maristan* (mental hospital), and had a chain put around his neck, and that was in the afternoon. When morning came and the *qadi* was presiding over court cases at the doorway of his house, he saw al-Waryaghli walking by, stamping the ground with his feet as was his custom. The *qadi* sent for the people of the *maristan* and asked them, 'Why did you let him go?' And they said, 'We know he is in the room!' They entered the room and found the chain as it was, still locked; and the *qadi* recognized him [as a saint] and resigned himself to the will of God, and he let him be.
>
> Al-Waryaghli did not ask anyone for anything, and of those who gave him something, sometimes he accepted it and sometimes he did not.
>
> He had a good voice, and sometimes he would sing *aroubi* songs[8] between the columns of the Qarawiyyin mosque loudly, until you would not wish to hear anything else, and the public agreed upon his *wilaya* [spiritual power, divine election] and that one could achieve *baraka* [God's blessing] through him, and many came to him with their problems and they derived benefit from him, from the signs which fell from his tongue.
>
> At the end of his life he never left a house in the al-Sagha neighbourhood, and people went to him there for visitation. They came with *sadaqat* [charity] and his *mubashir* [i.e. person who serves him, caretaker] takes the money, until he died in the house the eighteenth of Rajab in the year 1162... 'He died at the beginning of Rajab in the epidemic of the year 1163.' He was buried in the house in al-Sagha neighbourhood of the Adwa Fas al-Qarawiyyin, and a shrine was built upon him in a large garden, with decoration and embellishment, and there is a wooden *darbuz* upon his grave, and it is a famous place of visitation from which people take *baraka* until the present day.

The *majnun* stands in sharp contrast to the vast majority of Islamic saints in al-Kattani's compendium, whose piety, good works, noble conduct, and scholarship have inspired the community of believers. With the *majnun*'s bizarre behaviour, it is difficult to see him as an example of Islamic faith or the upholder of Islamic law in society, yet this is precisely our contention. Elements of al-Waryaghli's story show how the *majnun* restored God's law to men in their individual bodies and to the collective Islamic community.

8 *Aroubi*, i.e., 'in the dialect of the countryside'. This is a melody of vernacular Moroccan poetry, [*al-malhun*].

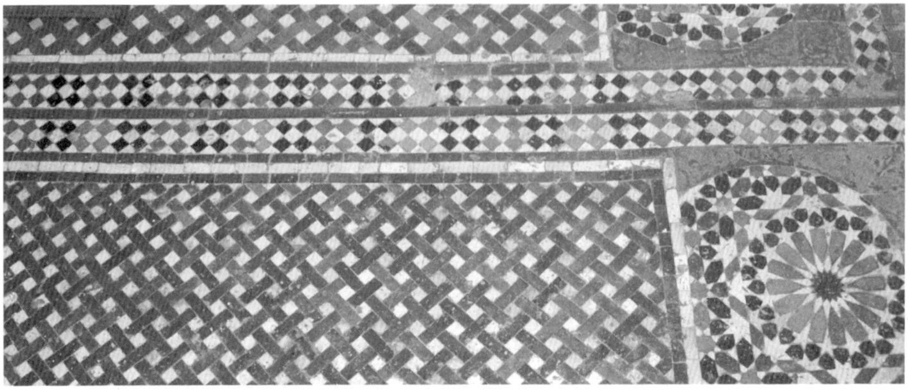

Graves in the floor of a saint shrine in Fez, Sidi 'al-Jilali'.
[Photo Ellen J. Amster]

First, al-Waryaghli demonstrates the egalitarianism of *ma'rifa*, God's election to receive knowledge of Him. With no blood relation to the Prophet Muhammad and no noble lineage, al-Waryaghli nevertheless receives knowledge of God; he is of sub-Saharan, African, non-Arab origins. A merchant, not a religious scholar, he walks away from ordinary life to exclusive devotion to God. His ordinariness illustrates the presence of God's Friends hidden among the common people and the democratic possibility of God's election.

Secondly, al-Waryaghli's body becomes an open channel for God's blessing, demonstrating the basic truth that the human body is a vessel for God. Unlike the Christian rejection of the flesh, the human body can contain God, according to the Prophetic *hadith qudsi*:

> God, He is most high, has said, 'Whoever treats a friend (*wali*) of mine as an enemy, takes the field against Me in battle. Nothing draws My servant near to Me like the performance of what I prescribe for him as religious duty. Then My servant continues to draw nearer to Me by supererogatory acts until I love him. So that, when I love him, I become the ear by which he hears, his eye by which he sees, his hand by which he grasps, and the foot by which he walks. Thus, by Me he hears; by Me he sees; by Me he grasps and by Me he walks. If he asks Me [for something] I certainly give it and if he seeks refuge with Me, indeed I protect him...[9]

For this reason, the buried bodies of saints shape the urban space of the city of Fez. A saint grave may grow into a shrine, a mosque, a Sufi lodge, or an entire city quarter. The body of Sidi Ahmad al-Shawi has become a city quarter, Sidi al-Khayyat is now a community mosque, and Sidi Qasim ibn Rahmun has be-

9 From the *Sahih* of al-Bukhari, cited in Homerin, 'Ibn Taimiya's *Al-Sufiya wa-al-Fuqara*'.

come a Sufi lodge.[10] The text of the *Salwa* is organized according to the physical locations of the saints, a cartographic imaginary different from a spatial map. The *Salwa* describes the city in a spiral, a pilgrimage route, beginning at the saint/sultan/founder of the Islamic state Idris II at the city centre and revolving out to the gardens and cemeteries at the city edge. As al-Kattani writes, the saints are geographical locations for God's blessing on earth, 'a refuge for those who fear, a place for sinners to find peace... doors to God on earth'.

The *majnun* al-Waryaghli illustrates a second quality of the Muslim saint: he shows the people how to live in God's community, 'God the Highest said, loving Me requires love of each other, loving Me requires cooperation, loving Me requires advising each other...'[11] The *majnun* breaks social norms, defies political authorities, and turns conventions upside down to show the people a hidden truth. As the Sufi al-Jazuli writes, 'The knowers of God (*al-'arifun*), are a folk who work righteousness...[thus] they are freed [from material constraints]... they die; when they die they come back [to God] and live [again]; when they live, they speak with the Living who never dies...'[12] Al-Waryaghli shows the superiority of God's will to man's earthly power, escaping conventional morality, the judge, and the chains of the insane asylum. The *majnun* Masa' al-Khayr al-Masmudi (d. 1705) shouted *masa' al-khayr*, 'good afternoon' to passer-by. 'The people understood this as a sign, that the people of goodness were going and goodness went with them, because in the afternoon the light is fading, and nothing remains after it but darkness.' If Ahmad ibn 'Umar al-Sharif al-Bahlul (d. 1655) gave a man a straw bag for vegetables, the recipient knew that he would soon die, 'all of his words were a sign'. Sidi Ahasayn al-Aqra' al-Fallusi (d. 1845) walked the markets barefoot; he 'had uncovering of secrets and news of invisible knowledge'.[13]

In several hagiographies, the *majnun* act as a living vehicle for God's will and His speech. In the palatine quarter of Fez, the sultan's son and delegate saw Masa' al-Khayr al-Masmudi dressed in rags with an entire cloak wrapped around his head. The prince ordered his guards to seize the strange man, but even restrained by soldiers, the saint confidently foretold the prince's own assassination:

> [Hafid] ordered that [the *wali*] be seized and brought to him... He asked, 'Are you really a *murabit*?' And al-Masmudi said, 'If God has said so!' And the son of the sultan said, 'And do you know God?' He said, 'Yes.' He said, 'By what do you know Him?' And he said, 'I know that He is

10 He was buried in a mill, and his companions bought a neighbouring house, added to it and made it a *zawiya* with *waqf*, a library, and a chandelier. Al-Kattani, *Salwat al-Anfas*, 108

11 Al-Tabrani, 'Al-Kathir', citing 'Ubada bin al-Samit, cited in al-Kattani, *Salwat al-Anfas*, 38.

12 Al-Jazuli, cited in Cornell, *Realm of the Saint*, 185.

13 Al-Kattani, *Salwat al-Anfas*, 293.

> the one who ordered you to be killed, and He offers no blood money [*dia*] for you!' And after that day Mawlay Hafid was assassinated in Fez Jdid, because he wanted to revolt against his father and [the sultan] knew this.[14]

In many hagiographies in the *Salwa*, the *majnun* appears to men in order to lead them from ordinary life to a life of devotion to God. The future great saint Sidi Muhammad ibn Amr Ibn Rahmun began his life as a humble weaver, until a *majnun* visited him daily to call him to God's service. The *majnun* declared, 'The people say, "You have done enough work producing this embroidery, so leave it for making another embroidery."' As a result, Ibn Rahmun 'entered the market of the next world, and it is the market of the mendicants [Sufis]'.[15]

The most puzzling is the repulsive, antinomian behaviour of the *majnun*, which Islamic physicians and legal authorities treated as mental illness.[16] Yet antinomianism arises from two aspects of sainthood: disappearance of the ego in union with God (*fana fi Allah*), and concealing one's election to prevent veneration. Several hagiographies describe union with God as a state of trance. Even respectable saints like the judge, professor, and legal scholar Sidi Muhammad al-Tawdi bin al-Talib al-Muri (d. 1794), seemed to be mentally ill when 'the greatest signs of election became apparent'; 'he had to lie down for longer than a year' and 'was in a spiritual state of absence'.[17] Another saint, whom Fez residents claimed appeared to them in dreams, deliberately behaved bizarrely to keep people away, 'he chose sometimes the road of self-blame to veil his actions and his words from the people of his time. And every *wali* has his veil [*hijab*].'[18]

In *God's Unruly Friends*, Ahmet Karamustafa argues that antinomian behaviour is a form of extreme piety intended to create a 'social wilderness' for the penitent, for 'social life inevitably distanced humanity from God'. [19] Total rejection of human culture is a critique of society and allows the *majnun* to conceal his spiritual state; public veneration would re-constitute his ego.[20] Al-Kattani describes several *majnun* as deliberately concealing their election,

14 Al-Kattani, *Salwat al-Anfas*, 157.

15 Ibid., 116.

16 Michael Dols notes that insanity was a legal disability in medieval Islamic law; the mad could not enter into contracts, marry, be a witness, or make wills. They were also not responsible for criminal offenses and were exempt from religious and social obligations, Dols, *Majnun*, Ch. 3 and 4. Karamustafa writes that the cultural elite of medieval Islamdom called dervishes riffraff, imposters, beggars, and swindlers, *God's Unruly Friends*, 5.

17 Al-Kattani, *Salwat al-Anfas*, 131.

18 Al-Kattani, speaking of Sidi Sliman bin 'Abd al-Hafid al-Kattani (d. 1857), in Ibid., 163.

19 Karamustafa, *God's Unruly Friends*.

20 Ibid., 30-32.

like Sidi 'Abd Allah bin Ibrahim al-Qalliz (d. 1682).[21] Al-Qalliz wore tattered, stained clothes and prayed in the mosque; when a man asked him for benediction, the *majnun* pushed him away angrily. The saint refused gifts and seemed to have lost his mind, though al-Kattani writes, 'it was customary for him to be excessive when concealing himself'.[22]

In these accounts, the body itself is a historical actor, an articulate subject whose miraculous responses validate the saint's election and special knowing (*ma'rifa*). Exceptional corporeal phenomena of the Islamic saint are in his own body (in the case of al-Waryaghli, vanishing from the shackles of an insane asylum), and in the bodies of others, either bringing God's mercy to the suffering by healing or punishing evildoers with pain, blindness, and disease. The Qur'an describes the human body as a location for God's signs (*ayat*)[23] and His obedient servant; the skin, hearing, and body parts will testify to God on the Day of Judgment, 'That day shall We set a seal on their mouths, but their hands will speak to Us and their feet bear witness to all that they did'(36:65). In *The Divine System for the Reform of the Human Kingdoms*, medieval Sufi scholar Muhya ad-Din Ibn al-'Arabi explains the relationship of body to body politic. As God appointed the human soul to be His Vice-Regent on earth, so He created the human body as a citadel for its residence. As a just ruler produces a harmonious city, so a just soul produces a harmonious body; an unjust soul will provoke the body's members to revolt. The healing powers of the Islamic saint thus depended upon a special epistemology, *ma'rifa*, and a theological understanding of the human body.

As Islam has no canonical Church to codify or regulate its miraculous phenomena, (indeed, the 'orthodox' Islamic scholars often rejected saintly miracles), the Moroccan public validated Islamic saints by acknowledging their miracles, visiting their bodies in life and after death, and narrating their miracle stories. Saintly knowing (*ma'rifa*) was thus potentially revolutionary, for it provided a means to challenge the sultans' political legitimacy and it was validated by the public. Sainthood often became political leadership in Moroccan history (the Almoravids, the Almohads, the Wazzaniyya, Ma' al-'Aynayn), and miracle-working saints have contended with the sultans for political power, created states or quasi states, governed territory, collected taxes, and negotiated trade agreements. It was this political aspect of Moroccan sainthood that first interested French visitors in the nineteenth century, as the European powers scrambled to colonize and exploit North Africa.

21 The following account is from Abu al-'Abbas Ahmad bin Muhammad bin Yaqub al Wallali, in his biography, 'Mubahith al-Anwar', from al-Kattani, *Salwat al-Anfas*, 119.

22 Al-Kattani, *Salwat al-Anfas*, 119-121.

23 The religious studies scholar Scott Kugle adapts the phenomenology of French theorist Maurice Merleau-Ponty to argue that the human body is 'the locus of the manifestation of God's names and attributes – a theophany of the highest order', Kugle, *Sufis and Saints' Bodies*, 29.

Madman, charlatan, or fetish man — French science and the *majnun*

The Islamic saints of interest to France in 1900 were not *majnun* but political leaders: Sufi leader 'Ma' al-'Aynayn' ('water of the two eyes') Qaldami, who led military jihad against the expansion of the French armies to Morocco from Mauritania, his son 'al-Hiba', who was declared sultan of Morocco by Marrakesh scholars in 1912, the saintly *sharif* of Wazzan 'Abd al-Salam, whom the French viewed as a 'prince' with an 'independent fiefdom' (and thus made a protégé of France), and the minor saints who led rural revolts against Sultans 'Abd al-Aziz (r. 1900-1907) and 'Abd al-Hafiz (r. 1908-1912). So bewildering was the Moroccan political landscape of 1905 that French military officer Edmond Ferry wrote, 'There is not one Morocco, but several Moroccos', each led by a person with 'a kind of blessing or divine power'; the Sultan himself was no more than a 'crowned [saint]'.[24] Officers of the Ministry of Foreign Affairs mention miracle stories in intelligence reports - Ma' al-'Aynayn was said to have brought a dead camel back to life, Al-Hiba was believed to metamorphose into a black cat to escape his enemies - but the French military dismissed such miracles as public hysteria or dubious propaganda.

Only the Durkheimian Edmond Doutté took seriously the miracle healing of the Muslim saints. The first editor of *L'Année sociologique* to specialize in Islam, Doutté was sent on five secret missions to Morocco by Affaires étrangères (1900-1905) to prepare France for the conquest of Morocco (1912). The key to Morocco's politics, he argued, lay in the thaumaturgy of the marabouts.[25] In his *Magie et religion dans l'Afrique du Nord* (1908), Doutté argued that Moroccans were primitives inhabiting a magical universe of demons, emotional projections of the savage mind. Observing that Muslim pilgrims rubbed their sick bodies with stones and placed them on a pile beside saint shrines, Doutté called this 'animist healing by magical transference'.[26] The marabout was thus no more than a superficially-Islamicized fetish - like the stone, he absorbed the tribe's maladies into his own body: 'The bodies of the saints become receptacles of the ills of the community.'[27] Thus, the Muslim crowds vying to touch the *sharif* of Wazzan or to swallow his saliva were not religious pilgrims but primitive, animist savages seeking relief from sickness.[28] Doutté concluded

24 Ferry, *La Réorganisation marocaine*.
25 Doutté, 'Notes sur l'islam maghribin'.
26 Id., *Les Tas de pierres sacrés*.
27 Id., *Merrâkech*, 107.
28 Id., *Les Tas de pierres sacrés*, 23.

that Muslims have a primitive *mentalité* defined by their religion of 'ritual, sacred, obligatory, and immutable character'. Because the categories of thought were irrational, Moroccan society had no science, law, free thought, or public morality.[29]

This illuminates the contention of Richard Keller, that Islam represented a 'space of insanity' for France.[30] In part, 'Islam as madness' arose from French colonial science in North Africa after 1880, where medicine and *sociologie*, 'sign and symptom', intertwined.[31] French doctors framed their understandings of Moroccan illness through a Durkheimian sociology of Islam, and French sociologists used traditional healing to prove Moroccan primitivism.[32] Qur'anic amulets, *jinn* possession, and saintly miracles all 'proved' Moroccan society to be irrational; medicine was used as the barometer of civilized thought. Doutté wrote, 'The doctor is at base a counter-sorcerer; the word T'ibb signifies magic as well as medicine; medicine is the daughter of magic. Even now, the doctor in North Africa is no more differentiated from the sorcerer than the malady from the djinn... the procedures to expel genies are beside therapeutic notes, rites of magic with the use of simples.'[33] French doctors criticized saint 'miracles' as iatrogenic and an obstacle to true medicine, as Alfred Bel wrote, '[The natives] take a bit of earth... impregnated with urine from this saintly man [al-Wazzani]... and carefully fill a wound that the French doctor didn't cure quickly enough.'[34]

On the eve of European colonialism, the *majnun* appears on the historical margins. European physicians, diplomats, and military officers often mention in passing that a *majnun* spit at them, threw things, or rushed at them with a weapon. After a *majnun* hit French consul Edouard Sourdeau in the face with a stick in 1820, Sultan Mawlay Sulayman wryly suggested the Christian injunction to turn the other cheek.[35] European travel accounts often include the 'colourful' *majnun*, his public nakedness, sexual libertinage, smoking, alcohol consumption, filthy hair, and bizarre speech.

Though marginal, the *majnun*'s holiness provided the French with ultimate evidence of Moroccan irrationality. 'The mad, in effect, the idiots, and those who pretend to be insane, (because there is reason to believe there are many fakers), are here surrounded by popular veneration... Dressed in rags, the [*majnun*] wander the streets of all native agglomerations, nourished by

29 Id., *Magie et religion dans l'Afrique du Nord*, 7-8.
30 Keller, *Colonial Madness*, 1-10.
31 Amster, *Medicine and the Saints*, Chapter 2.
32 Ibid., 52.
33 Doutté, *Magie et religion dans l'Afrique du Nord*, 35-36.
34 Cited in Rivet, *Lyautey et l'institution du protectorat*, II, 240. Women in Tangier visited the Wazzani to cure sterility, Service Historique de l'Armée de Terre (hereafter SHAT), Carton 3H1: Marois, 'Relation d'un voyage au Maroc: Ambassade française, mars-avril 1877'.
35 Doutté, 'Notes sur l'islam maghribin', 294.

the public charity.'[36] That Moroccans should seek cure from the mad, and the ravings of the mentally ill should be venerated as missives from God, simply revealed that Islam itself was a form of madness. This madness, the primitivism of the savage mind, pervaded Moroccan society: 'Sacred trees, epileptic madmen [*majnun*], and shrines' are all called 'marabout', observed Doutté, thus marabout really signifies 'instrument of healing'.[37]

After 1900, many French physicians identified Islamic sainthood and *jinn* beliefs as the antithesis of science and civilization. The first director of native health for French Morocco, Mauran, described *jinn* possession and Sufi trance (*hadra*) as 'pathology, delirium, and contagion'. 'These exhibitions disgust me profoundly and I flee them... I accuse them of perpetuating fanaticism and ignorance, of capturing the soul of the people, preventing them from thinking... which drags them down to the worst misery and servitude.'[38] Physician Emile Mauchamp argued that French hygiene would modernize Morocco, but 'before one dreams of rebuilding this society on the bases of modern progress... Let us denounce the enemies of human reason', the marabouts and the sorcerers.[39] Because Moroccans believed *jinn* to be the cause of fevers, paralysis, attacks of the nerves, convulsions, haemorrhages, and eye maladies,[40] saints fooled the people with their phoney miraculous cures. '[The saint/sorcerer's] prestige reflects the mentality of his dupes in this country, where at every step one fears to offend or step on a devil.'[41] French imperialists proposed positivist medicine as the path for liberating the Moroccan and constituting him as a rational subject.

These examples demonstrate how French colonialism in Morocco was an epistemological struggle, a war of positivism against Sufi Islam to heal and thus define the human being.[42] French physicians and *sociologues* rejected Sufi epistemology (*ma'rifa*) entirely - when presented with a Sufi Sanusiyya text depicting the stages of the soul's development, Doutté scoffed: 'This sounds like Saint Theresa and the seven mystical *chateaux*. It is nothing but a morbid psychological state described by M. Ribot in his book on maladies of attention.'[43] In part, these doctors imagined themselves joining a much older struggle against religion and the occult; Mauchamp compared Moroccan healing to the Albiginian heresies, the grotto of Lourdes, and folk practices of Bre-

36 Doutté, 'Notes sur l'islam maghribin'.
37 Ibid., 32.
38 Mauran, *La Société marocaine*, 214-218.
39 Mauchamp, *La Sorcellerie au Maroc*, 100 and 203.
40 Ibid., 189.
41 Ibid., 201.
42 Amster, *Medicine and the Saints*, Introduction.
43 Doutté, *L'Islam algérien en l'an 1900*, 64.

ton peasants.[44] But he also suggests a uniquely neurotic 'Muslim' physiognomy, 'excessively impressionable, vibrating, passionate... moved to the extreme by rhythm, which address the nerves rather than the intelligence... *The Arab is a voluptueux*, an Oriental, a Semite: perfumes, music, parties, slaves; all is voluptuary...'[45] French doctors pathologized Islamic mystical phenomena as hysteria or neurosis, especially *jinn* possession. The *jinn*-possessed 'Muslim madman' found scientific elaboration as a type in the asylums of Dr Antoine Porot, the architect of French psychiatric assistance in North Africa and founder of the 'Algiers School' of North African psychiatry.[46]

The belief in *jinn* possession, and the *majnun* himself, constituted the irreducible difference between French and Moroccan ideas of reality, as Keller argues: 'For many colonial physicians, belief in the *jnun* and their actions constituted a sign of pathological difference that played a central role in shaping mental illness.'[47] French denial of Islamic epistemology reduced the Muslim to an entirely corporeal existence, one in which there could be no transcendence, only neurological symptoms and pathologies. Yet as we have seen, French colonial sciences pathologized Islam itself.[48] As Keller has suggested, the psychiatric construction of the 'Muslim madman' as a violent, fundamentally irrational figure unassimilable to civilization found a long life in French literature and film; he often came to represent the North African Muslim generally, informing even debates about Muslim immigration to France.[49]

Madman and heretic, Moroccan Islamic modernity and the *majnun*

French positive science also deeply influenced the Moroccan nationalist movement (1930-1956), which led Moroccan nationalists to reject the *majnun* and *jinn* possession as intellectual backwardness and heresy. Even as nationalists across North Africa attacked France for the hypocrisy of its civilizing mission, they applied French definitions of sovereignty, citizenship, and scientific modernity to Moroccan society. The Moroccan body, and exceptional corporeal phenomena in general, were consequently understood through French science by Moroccans in independent Morocco.

44 Mauchamp, *La Sorcellerie au Maroc*, 96. Interestingly, a critic of modernity and positivism in metropolitan France like René Guénon abandoned spiritism, occultism, and theosophy as invalid, but turned to Sufism as a source of true enlightenment. Guénon joined a Sufi order in 1911 and finally moved to Cairo in the 1930s. Monroe, *Laboratories of Faith*.

45 Mauchamp, *La Sorcellerie au Maroc*, 77.

46 Keller, *Colonial Madness*, Chapter 2.

47 Ibid., 114.

48 Ibid., 9.

49 Ibid., 208-226.

Moroccan history was re-imagined by the nationalists to exclude the saints; the royal dynastic chronicle *Kitab al-Istiqsa' li akhbar duwwal al-maghrib al-aqsa* of Ahmad Khalid al-Nasiri was adopted as the official narrative of Moroccan history, and the saint-centred, miraculous *Salwat al-Anfas* of al-Kattani was rejected. Moroccan saints like Muhammad al-Jazuli were recrafted as 'proto-nationalists' who had paved the way for nationalism by creating a 'religion of the people'. In this way, saints, sainthood, and saintly knowing (*ma'rifa*) were erased from the narrative of Morocco's history and replaced by a national and dynastic model of sovereignty.[50]

Nationalists also defined the relationship of the state to the citizen's body, a necessity forced by the public health crises of 1937-1956. Nationalists agreed that Moroccan hunger, epidemics, and poverty were the result of 'twenty-five years of exploitation of the native to the benefit of the colonizer',[51] but they embraced French biomedicine as the right of the Moroccan citizen and the cornerstone of the Moroccan nation. The newspaper *Al Hayat* argued that training Moroccan doctors was essential 'to ensure the free and independent life of the nation', and nationalists called for modern (French) medicine and pharmacy to be taught in a new, European-style university.[52]

By contrast, nationalists attacked Muslim saint healing as heretical, savage, and unscientific. The 1935 Congress of North African Muslim Students resolved that 'true scientific culture' must be inculcated 'into the brains of North-African children' to combat 'women's ignorance, heretical practices, and the ignorance of religion'.[53] The nationalist leader 'Allal Al-Fassi and scholars at the Qarawiyyin university petitioned the sultan to outlaw yearly celebrations for the saints, where 'heterodox practices' perpetuated 'popular ignorance of pure and noble Islam'. *Al Alam* complained: '[The people] do not understand the necessity of medical care and prevention... [Most] believe in superstition, magic and the intervention of angels and Satan in illness and cure.' The magical, emotional, *jinn*-possessed body of the *majnun* was a public embarrassment; the horrified nationalist al-Wazzani protested that European filmmakers recorded the *jinn*-possessed 'as if it were the present style in our country and defined the evolutionary social stage of our people'. He demanded: 'Rather, one should show the other Morocco, the modern Morocco, of a new generation.'[54]

Moroccan nationalism had adopted the Islamic modernist thought (*salafiyya*) of Egypt and the Levant, a movement of the late nineteenth century to reconcile Islam with positivism. A new episteme changed Moroccan

50 Amster, *Medicine and the Saints*, Chapter 6.
51 SHAT, Carton 3H1423: 'Allal al-Fasi in *Al Maghrib*, 16 April 1937.
52 Ibid.: *Al Hayat*, 11 April 1935.
53 SHAT: Carton 3H1423.
54 Muhammad al-Wazzani, from *L'Action du peuple*, cited in Spadola, 'The Scandal of Ecstasy'.

political legitimacy, for 'questions of epistemology are also questions of social order'.[55] The Moroccan modernists attacked the *majnun* and saint healing as backward, the oppression of the credulous by self-serving charlatans and heretics. The fighting saints of the nineteenth century, like the Mahdi of Sudan and 'Abd al-Qadir in Algeria, largely disappeared from the Islamic world in the twentieth century, replaced by modernist nationalists and the centralized state. The *majnun* became socially marginal in Morocco, even as he entered cultural metonymy in France - two sides of the same engagement of French positivism with Islam.

Conclusion

The example of the *majnun* as healer shows the paradigmatic importance of epistemology to ways of interpreting the human body and its exceptional corporeal phenomena. In French Morocco, we find a purely materialist conception of the body from French positivism confronting a Qur'anic and Sufi phenomenology of the body. For French positivism, corporeal phenomena associated with Moroccan saint healing could only be neurological or neurotic phenomena. The positivist epistemological frame did not allow for seeing the human body as a vessel for God, or as an articulate creation of God which testified directly to Him. Rather than a healer of Islamic society, the *majnun* was understood by the French as a patient, a madman, and a suffering soul who needed rational medical care.

For the French colonizer, Moroccan veneration of the *majnun* as a saintly healer demonstrated a savage understanding of the natural world, one which pervaded Islamic society and proved the difference between the primitive and the civilized. To colonize Morocco, French administrators proposed to study, catalogue, and scientifically manage the primitive Moroccan *mentalité* through French colonial governance. The *majnun* himself was often incarcerated in the new French insane asylums of North Africa, where Dr Antoine Porot and his disciples elaborated a 'Muslim madman', an ethnopsychiatric type who embodied the irrationality of Islam and the supposed hypersensitivity of the Arab nervous system. Before colonialism, the *majnun* had been marginal to Islamic hagiography and European visitors. After French conquest, the *majnun* became central, perhaps emblematic of Morocco to French colonial science, a fundamentally irrational Islamic figure whose unassimilable character opposed Western civilization.

The *majnun* sheds light on larger questions of the body as a site for colonial modernity, epistemology, and subjectivity. In the Moroccan nationalist rejection of the *majnun*, we find a larger Islamic modernist *salafi* internali-

55 Latour, *We Have Never Been Modern*, 15-16.

zation of France as the model of scientific modernity. In embracing French science as an unquestioned good, Islamic modernists unconsciously ingested French positivism as the structuring epistemology for reality, absorbing the positivist repugnance for Sufi forms of knowledge. As the body remains the frame of individual subjectivity, we also find the incomplete victory of positive nationalism in Morocco. Traditional healing has not disappeared; Moroccan patients yet integrate shrine visitation, midwives, and traditional apothecaries with biomedicine in their 'quest for therapy'.[56] Medical pluralism suggests a persistence of Sufi epistemologies in the body. 'You will take bread (*baraka*, blessing) from Fez', said the 95 year old lady whose *majnun* father is described at the beginning of this piece, 'You will take bread (*khobz)* back to America, to your family and your life there.' And so I have.

56 Janzen, *The Quest for Therapy in Lower Zaire.*

EXPERIENCING RELIGION AND MEDICINE

MARIAN APPARITION AND VICTIM SOULS IN PORTUGAL, 1910-1950*

TIAGO PIRES MARQUES

For all the cultural wars of the positivist era, when faced with the otherness of the mad and the mystic, theology and psychiatry have held rather more in common than both would perhaps like to admit. In continental Catholic Europe, for example, renowned and leading representatives of psychiatry attempted to establish the doctrine that the contents of delusions were neither relevant nor important to the diagnosis. Nevertheless, psychiatric vignettes abounded with details on the actual experience of 'being mad'. Symmetrically, Catholic theologians may have adhered to the traditional view that only conformity between the spiritual results of mystical experiences and Vatican theology would enable them to assert the authenticity of the mystic; however, they had long since resorted to doctors in order to rule out possible physical and psychological causes of phenomena observed.[1]

Nevertheless, these intersections have rarely been studied from the perspective of the ways in which the dynamic relationship between scientific and religious epistemologies interferes with the actual experiences. This article argues that, in the first few decades of the twentieth century, these intersections underwent significant historical changes. More concretely, it builds on the idea that medical knowledge was interwoven with religious experience

* The author gratefully acknowledges the financial support of the exploratory project 'The Fabric of Mental Health. Medical Power, Secularity, and the Psychotherapeutic Field in Portugal (1940s-1990s)', funded by the Portuguese Foundation for Science and Technology (FCT). The author would like to thank the reviewers for their helpful comments for the improvement of this manuscript.

1 Marques, 'Mystique, politique et maladie mentale', 37-74.

which, in turn, actualized or helped displace certain scientific themes. Rather than a conflict between the medical and religious epistemologies, this analysis finds that some Catholic milieus adapted well to the rationalist requirements of modernity by both constructing hybrid epistemologies and creating or emphasizing new forms of ascertaining the authenticity and credibility of extraordinary or 'miraculous' religious forms.

The Marian apparitions of Fátima in 1917 and the case of the Blessed Alexandrina of Balasar (1904-1955) provide us with material rich in suggestions as to the mutual interferences between changing experiences of religious symbols and emotions and developments and lay appropriations of psychiatry. While Fátima, one of the most successful Marian sanctuaries in the world, is widely known, Alexandrina's story deserves a brief introduction. Born in Balasar, a small, rural village in the Northwest of Portugal, Alexandrina Maria da Costa belongs to the Catholic mystical tradition of so-called 'victims souls', which was fairly common in Portugal in the nineteenth and twentieth centuries.[2] As a result of illness, and similar to other contemporary mystics such as Therese Neumann (1898-1962) and Marthe Robin (1902-1981), Alexandrina became bedridden at an early age. In her writings, she describes her life as one of unremitting physical and moral pain, which she eventually offered up to God in atonement for the sins of humankind. By the time of her death, she was viewed locally as a saint. However, her sainthood was highly controversial during her lifetime and while she continued to be locally remembered due to a small group of enthusiastic supporters, Alexandrina soon lost credibility among the ecclesiastical authorities. Under Pope John Paul II, however, her cause was revived, culminating in her beatification in 2004.

Medical observations play a role in both cases as a means of contesting and/or confirming their validity. In each case, medical references were applied differently, so that we can distinguish two different epistemologies of religious experience within the same Catholic and cultural universe. Thus, the primary objective of this article is to provide an account of this historical cohabitation as well as competition between different experiential and epistemological configurations. We pay particular attention to the mechanisms employed to enhance credibility in authoritative discourses and reports on embodied experiences.

2 For the Portuguese case, see: Cabral, *Sons of Adam, Daughters of Eve*, 226-232; on victim soul spirituality elsewhere, see: Kane, 'She offered herself up'.

Marian apparitions

Ever since 1916, when some children from Fátima first said they had seen a 'white figure', rumours abounded, which were subsequently echoed in the first documents that appeared in the wake of the apparitions.[3] In effect, the first narratives reflect a childish and becharmed ambience, the colour of which would eventually fade during the exhaustive theological questioning of Father Manuel Formigão, taking place from late September 1917 onwards. Lúcia told the Fátima parish priest, Father Manuel Marques Ferreira, that she had seen the 'Lady' rise up out of the holm oak grove and head heavenwards. Going into detail, the figure had its 'toes bunched up and the body already hidden'.[4] To the same parish priest, Jacinta affirmed as to having seen the Lady in the church where she was taught to 'pray the beads (the rosary)'. On another occasion, she saw her at night, over the loft entranceway and a third time beneath the table: 'Look... can't you see the Lady, who I saw up there, now down below?!.... Look!!!', Jacinta exclaimed to her mother.[5] The family home and the celestial worlds had suddenly begun communicating in both stories, although in different ways. In the case of Lúcia, through an opening in the vaulted ceiling through which a feminine entity passed with whom she was able to converse. In the case of Jacinta, the vision was shared at certain moments by Lúcia and Francisco, while the image appeared to her at other moments in private and sometimes in unexpected places, such as the loft and beneath the table.

This apparition was one of a series of extraordinary religious events in Portugal in the aftermath of the aggressively secularist regime of the First Republic (1910-1926). Indeed, for the years 1916 and 1917 alone, there were six other sites with apparitions reported, all of which eventually fell into oblivion. In the next three sections, we look at the diversity of elements that proved crucial to the credibility of Fátima.[6]

Making-up a credible body

Let us examine, more in detail, the documents reporting the interrogations of the seers. Just after the first apparition, the parish vicar asked Lucia and the other two children to obey the lady and go to the site, after which they should return and report to him what they had seen. He explicitly declared that, to avoid malicious interpretations, he would be silent on what to ask the Lady.

3 The documents assembled in Documentação Crítica de Fátima are referred to by the abbreviation DCF. Mother of Lúcia. Transcript, DCF, I, 83; Questioning by Manuel Nunes Formigão, DCF, I, 150.

4 Questioning of the vicar of Fátima, DCF, I, 16.

5 'Processo paroquial de Fátima', DCF, I, 270.

6 Carvalho, *Os Levantes da República*, 308-309 and 317-329.

He would retain a neutral position and focus only on writing down Lúcia's statements. Set in a descriptive and purportedly objective style, in which only the voices of Lucia and that of the Lady are conveyed in direct speech, these notes convey the image of a 'Lady' descending from the tree after an atmospheric signal (often lightening) and almost always at noon. Lucia sees and hears what the Lady says, while Francisco and Jacinta can see her but they cannot hear her. The first apparition happens only to the children, while the following ones (as in Lourdes) attracted increasing numbers of people from the region. Joining the apparition site in hope of seeing the Lady, they testified the children's pious behaviour. In one apparition, the still unidentified Lady eventually delivers a message about the duration of the on-going World War. However, by far the most recurrent topic in the reported dialogue between the seer and the priest concerns the Lady's outfit. Next to nothing is said about her face, expression and beauty: asked on one occasion whether the Lady was smiling or weeping, Lucia answered 'neither'. Apparently no signs of emotions were identifiable in her expression. Furthermore, from the outset, it also becomes clear that the Lady is a healer or at least has the power of recommending the healing of the sick, with requests and offers (including money) piling up ever since the second apparition.[7]

In late September 1917, between the fifth and the sixth and last apparition, Father Formigão stepped onto Fatima's scene. He was a different kind of priestly figure. Returning from Rome where he had studied theology and canonical law, he had spent time in Lourdes where – as stated in his own memoir – he promised Our Lady to make the spreading of her cult his mission. Indeed, in the years following the apparitions, he became the driving force behind the expansion of Fatima.[8] The author of the first apologetic books on the apparitions, published in 1921, he mediated between the children, local priests and notables as well as the Church's higher hierarchy. This crucial role was formally recognized as he led the canonical commission charged with validating the events. The commission report, a crucial document for the official approval of the cult, was published in 1930, already into the formative years of the conservative and dictatorial regime known as the Estado Novo ('New State').

Father Formigão began his interrogation of the seers – whom he shall soon be calling the 'shepherds' – in late September 1917. His notes, writing style and interrogation technique are very different from those of the local priest: literary and extensively corrected, he worked as if some detective in search of contradictions, whether factual or doctrinal. In a word, he worked as an old style inquisitor. No longer a supposedly objective transcription of the seers' impressions, his notes reflect this detailed and repetitive form of in-

7 Questioning of the vicar of Fátima, DCF, I, 11-12.
8 Torgal, *O Sol bailou ao Meio-Dia*.

quiry. As opposed to both the seers and the local priest, he immediately identified the lady as Our Lady, the Blessed Virgin Mary Mother of Jesus. However, he was concerned with some troubling details that did not fit the image of Our Lady: the earrings, the socks, the length of the skirt, even the inexpressive features of the Lady's face, who neither wept as in La Salette nor smiled as in Lourdes. The short skirt proved particularly alarming: this might actually even constitute a sign that what the children took for a heavenly entity was in fact the devil in disguise.

After a few more interrogations about these details, he eventually obtained a more suitable image of the Lady. Indeed, Lúcia changed her version and acquiesced that the mantle did indeed cover the whole body, including the head, and that no earrings could have been seen. The problem of the white socks was solved in a particularly graceful manner: 'Are you sure that what you took for white socks weren't instead her bare feet, so white and glowing that you were misled in your vision?', he asked.[9] Lucia agreed. Father Formigão also insisted on the matter of the Lady's beauty, asking the seers to compare her with a pretty girl who was passing by. Lucia added that the Lady was more beautiful than any other person she had seen.[10]

Before the last and most important apparition, in which the Lady would finally reveal her identity and the reason for her presence in Fátima, the sessions spent questioning Lúcia had built up an image of the Lady's body suitable to identification with that of 'Our Lady'. In the canonical report, the image's description was stabilized as follows:

> The Apparition looked no more than 18 years old. Her dress was of the purest snowy white, just as the mantle, edged with gold, covered her head and most of her body. The face, showing a faultless nobility of lines and with a supernatural and divine indescribable touch, was serene and serious as if veiled by a light shadow of sadness. From her hands, held together at the height of her chest, a beautiful rosary was suspended, finishing in a cross and covered with beads of stoat-fur whiteness that resembled pearls. From the whole figure, surrounded by a shining brighter than the sun, beams of light irradiated, especially from the face, of a beauty impossible to describe and incomparably superior to human beauty.[11]

9 Questioning by Dr Manuel Nunes Formigão, DCF, I, 49.
10 Ibid., 47.
11 'Processo Canónico Diocesano', DCF, II, 162.

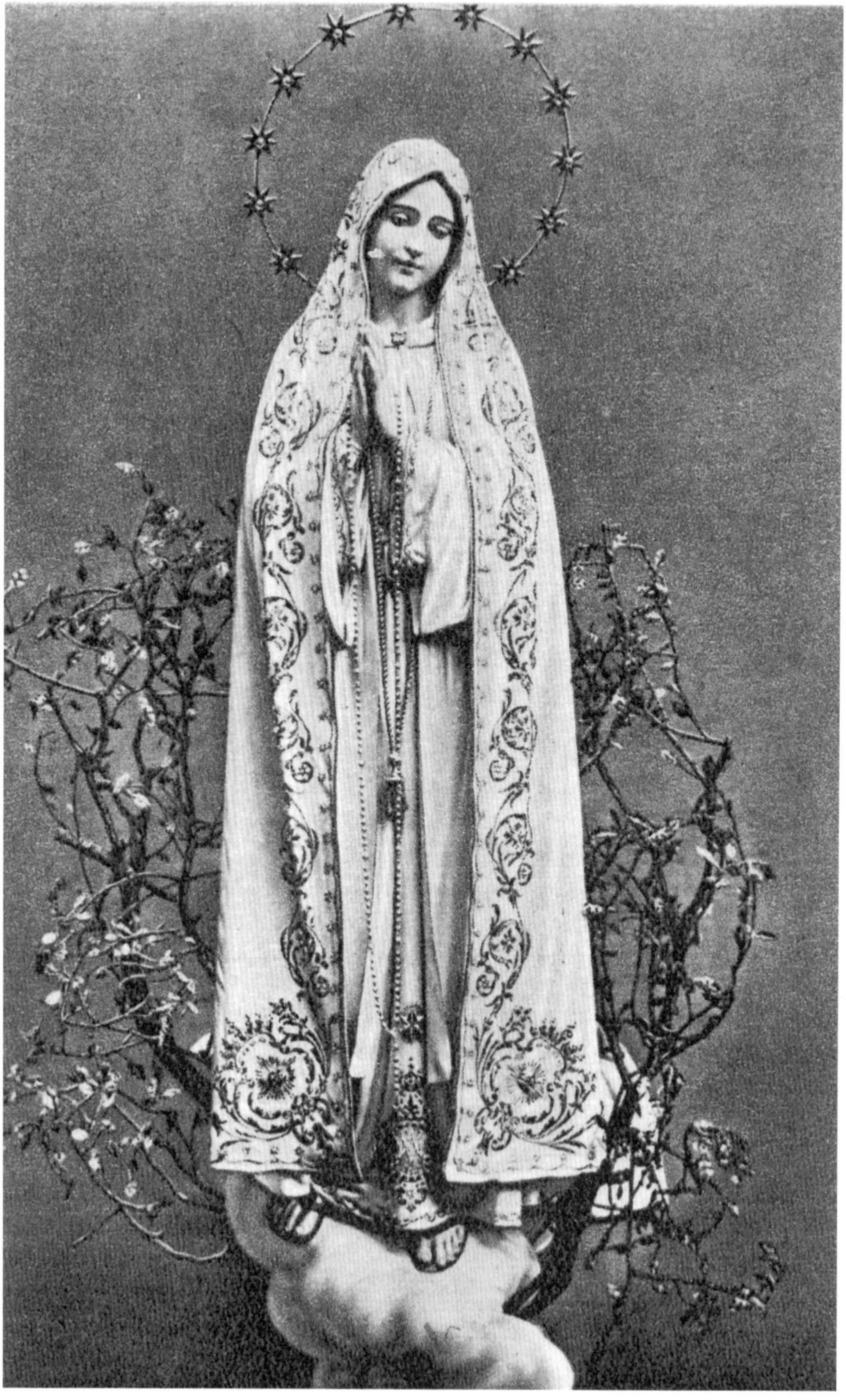

Devotional printed image of Our Lady of Fatima. Date unknown (first encountered for the year 1939). [*Private collection*]

The heavenly body of Fátima was no longer the fuzzy image of a 'Lady'. It had objectively become the body of Our Lady.[12]

A breach in the laws of nature

The apparition of 13 October gathered thousands of pilgrims from all classes and ages – 40,000 to 50,000 according to the vicar. This apparition differed significantly from the others. The Lady again descended from the sky to the tree, announced the end of the war that very day and begged for the construction of a chapel in honour of the Rosary, insisting that the people should pray the Rosary. She then went back up to the sky and after losing sight of her, Lúcia saw, to the left of the sun, Saint Joseph holding the Infant Jesus in one hand and blessing the crowd with the other. The Infant Jesus, says the priest's report, was dressed in red. To the right of the sun, Our Lady then reappeared, also dressed in red and with a blue mantle covering her head. This vision vanished before another image formed in the sky, that of 'Our Lord' (Jesus Christ), visible only from the waist up, and dressed in white. Next to Our Lord, on his right side, Our Lady again appeared, this time dressed in white but with the blue mantle again covering her head. The vicar states that while Lucia was seeing these 'representations', the crowd shouted: 'Look... look... it is so beautiful!!'[13]

This was the grand finale to a pre-announced series of apparitions and the last to be covered by the press. A photographer of a national periodical wrote a piece on the apparitions, illustrated by photos of the crowd showing ecstatic faces staring at the sky. According to their testimonies, they neither saw any Lady, whether in red or in white, nor the Infant Jesus, nor Saint Joseph.[14] However, they did see something quite spectacular: the sun is said to have changed colour several times and to have turned around on itself, giving the impression that it would crush against the earth. This became known as the 'miracle of the sun' and is a key component of the Fatima narrative. The dance of the sun on that rainy day, breaching the laws of nature, stood for the authenticity of the seers' reports.

12 David Morgan rightly emphasizes the importance of the children's initial misrecognition of Our Lady to assert the authenticity of Fatima and other modern apparitions. For a more developed account of the relations between description of the viewed image, recognition and formation of devotional images of Our Lady of Fatima, see Morgan, *The Embodied Eye*, 193-202.

13 'Processo paroquial de Fátima', DCF, I, 268.

14 Ibid., 267-268.

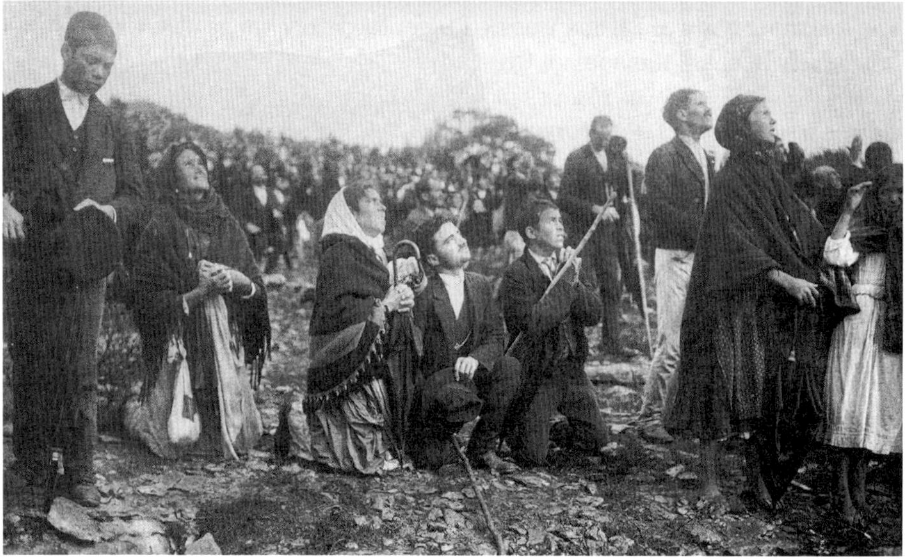

People standing staring at the sun: 'Several aspects of the people kneeling down and praying at the moment when they viewed the sun and the phenomenon that much impressed the crowd'.
[lustração Portuguesa. *Lisbon, 2 (160), 29 October 1917, 353*]

The belief process

Testimonies of the events of 13 October converged into the idea that something 'extraordinary' happened that day. Yet, even among devout Catholics the nature of the events was not clear. Carlos de Azevedo Mendes, a young notable of the region, doctor in law from Coimbra, is a particularly valuable witness. Driven to Fátima by curiosity in early September that year, he had interrogated the seers and testified also to the September's apparition. Although he was very much conquered by the simplicity of the children and the authenticity of the people's devotion, and also prone to consider that something extraordinary was happening, he did not venture to identify the extraordinary events as a Marian apparition. A letter to a brother, following the events of 13 October (the day of the 'sun miracle'), proves elucidative of the process of belief formation. First, he mentioned the impression of the extraordinary, namely through participation in a collective religious fervour and the feeling of beauty. However, not even the solar phenomenon sufficed to render the apparition certain. True, 'the atmospheric signals' were impressive and had never before been seen. Azevedo Mendes nevertheless asked (twice): were these phenomena natural? The question pointed to the possibility of a natural explanation. However, 'what matters... nobody had experienced them before...' It was important that the children had been announcing for six months that there would be 'a signal that would make everybody believe that the Lady truly did appear'. And he immediately added: 'It was beautiful to see those thousands of believers on that occasion!!'[15]

Aesthetic emotions came bound up with a rational argument. Thus, Azevedo Mendes started to make qualifications in the levels of extraordinariness of the events: the phenomena were forecast beforehand, and, in corroboration, these phenomena – even if merely natural – were not known to anybody. The 'miracle of the sun' was not, however, an apparition itself, nor a *proof* of the apparition, but rather a *signal* of the authenticity of the experience of the witnesses. From a purely intellectual and rational point of view, it was also necessary to account for the war not ending on that day, as had been announced by Lúcia. Azevedo Mendes refers to the fact, but does not qualify it as an element of counter-evidence. Among the signals produced in Fátima, Azevedo Mendes gathered emotions linked to a sense of beauty and innocence, relegating the rational arguments to secondary importance.[16]

The final paragraph of the letter to his brother contains an exercise in introspection. Azevedo Mendes explicitly analysed the structure of his belief, which we may summarise in the table below.

Ontological statute of the events	Form of belief
1. Extraordinary	Experience and rumours
2. Supernatural	Intimate conviction
3. Miraculous/Marian apparition	Suspended adhesion*

* 'Will there be a miracle?... I shall retain my own expectations until the Church issues its ruling and more especially because I have heard said that they are proceeding with an inquiry; however, in my intimacy, I have the extremely strong conviction that in all of the case of Fátima there is something of the supernatural' [My translation from Portuguese]. Letter by Dr. Carlos de Azevedo Mendes to one of his brothers, November 1917, DCF, I, 398.

In summary, the children were the vehicle for a synthesis of the extraordinary with the supernatural, but not for the identification of the 'Lady' with 'Our Lady'. Furthermore, this example also suggests that the making of this connection between the extraordinary and the supernatural required sharing of the belief by an extended circle of believers from different social classes.[17] On the side of the bourgeois or the rural nobility, these differences in a first instance played out through an observational and objective distancing, which was transformed into affective adhesion due to the 'rusticity' and 'simplicity' of the seers. This is the passage in which Azevedo Mendes established what he called an 'intimate conviction', still not yet shared but susceptible to entering the social space of belief. In turn, in the eyes of the rural population, the belief and adhesion of these members of the educated classes of landowners, sala-

15 Letter by Dr Carlos de Azevedo Mendes to one of his brothers, November 1917, DCF I, 397.
16 On the role of aesthetic emotions in processes of belief, see Tunhas, 'Três tipos de crenças', 134.
17 Marques, 'Extraordinary Order'.

ried employees and prestigious liberal professions (e.g. doctors and lawyers) collectively served as a guarantee of their veracity. Azevedo Mendes described a short episode in a letter to his future wife: on returning to his home near Fátima, his servants repeatedly asked whether it was true what one was saying about the apparitions.[18] If their master, a graduate of Coimbra and a figure revered for his knowledge, believed, then why would they not also believe? Other city-dwellers who travelled to Fátima, on 13 October, sometimes accompanied by their servants, reported their journey. These accounts present similar emotional responses to the observed religious fervour.[19]

Believable subjects

For all the affection that the seers inspired, proof of their sincerity remained insufficient for a validation of the religious nature of these events. Besides all the theological matters, modern psychiatry had already taught that many mentally ill people sincerely report their own visions, which ought to be considered delusions or hallucinations. Father Formigão foresaw this objection and delivered careful analysis that drew on the psychiatric vocabulary of his time. This was already the case in his first apologetic writing on Fatima, as early as November 1917, in a chapter called 'The sincerity of the seers and the truth of their declarations'. It remained a concern in his later canonical report. In both documents, he emphasized the apparently perfect 'physical and moral normalcy' of the seers. He then proceeded to distinguish between the question of the sincerity of the seers, which was not to be doubted on account of their moral behaviour as well as the integrity of their families, and the possibility of mental illness. The latter issue deserved detailed reasoning through a set of parameters defined along two axes: 1) the nature and predisposition of the seers; and 2) the quality of the hallucinations compared to authentic visions.[20]

On the first parameter, he argued that in order to be victim of 'nervous hallucinations', one has to be previously characterized as of a 'nervous nature'. However, none of the children had any such nature: they had never even been ill. In addition, they were not pensive or meditative; on the contrary, they were naturally joyful and expansive. Their ignorance in matters of religious education was also a guarantee that they had not been victim of 'religious excitation'. Such ignorance was otherwise proven by Lúcia's declaration that the Lady was more powerful than God Himself. Formigão then systematically compared the hallucinations of women in psychiatric hospitals with these visions. At this point, he observed that children rarely hallucinate and that hallucinations are typical of older women, whom he calls 'ill persons with

18 Letter from Azevedo Mendes to his future wife, 8 September 1917, DCF, I, 393.
19 DCF, III.
20 DCF, II, 164-172.

impaired brains'. These women are predisposed to the manifestations of their illness, which are a product of long processes that the priest then contrasts with the idyllic infancy of these children in the mountains.[21]

The second parameter was further divided into verifying phenomena before, during and after the visions. The visions of Fatima's seers came after a prophecy, whereas hallucinations do not follow prophecies. Hallucinating persons, the priest argued, display an absolute certainty in the reality of what they see as their organisms produce the vision. In contrast, the seers were docile and obedient. The setting also played a role in distinguishing between the two phenomena: whereas hallucinations are only produced under certain circumstances, visions may happen in different circumstances. This was the case in Fatima where the Lady was seen in different situations and among crowds, a factor the priest took as proof that such visions were produced by an outside reality, totally independent from the seer. He made, moreover, a distinction between the effects of the two types of phenomena: 'hallucinating hysterical women' retained vague memories of the hallucination; in contrast, authentic visions had impressively detailed characteristics. Proof of that lay in the seer's account of the Lady's outfit. Lastly, in the Catholic tradition the authenticity of a mystical experience is observed in its fruits. Hallucinations are viewed as sterile and morbid in their effects, and the hallucinating individual as proud, irritable and undisciplined. Authentic visions, on the contrary, produce virtuous persons, miracles, healings and strengthen the faith of the crowds. Lucia remained joyful and expansive even after entering religious life. Furthermore, there was, to cap it all, the 'miracle of the sun' to stand as irrefutable proof of the truth of the apparitions.

In sum, the canonical commission articulated psychiatric concepts and mobilized a set of counter-arguments to undermine explanations of the phenomena on pathological grounds. In a sense, these arguments formed a system of counter-symptoms that left a space open for divine signs to be plausible and meaningful. As far as psychiatry was concerned, the 'hysterical woman' had become the typical counter-example of authentic religious experiences.

Victim souls

Alexandrina, like other traditional mystical women, could not rely on what we can call the *barrier of counter-symptoms*. She had been sick in her childhood and bed-ridden all her life. In addition, her spiritual accounts, deeply rooted in the traditional model of female sainthood, did not emphasize joy but instead expressed the theme of suffering, which had become highly suspicious

21 DCF, II, 168 and 170.

in modern times.[22] Many passages in her writings testify to her sufferings, on the brink of abjection:

> 20 October 1940
>
> At the end of April 1937, I went through a great crisis that took me to death's door. I began throwing up day and night, holding nothing in my stomach. In the first few days, I was struck with profound prostration. I recognized nobody, I felt neither hunger nor thirst. The abbot read the prayers of agony three times. I only recall a few words he said on one of those occasions. I heard screams but I didn't think I died since my physical state wouldn't allow me to. [...]
>
> It was a terrifying tribulation, which got repeated over and over. I had the most furious attacks twice a day, at 9 or 10 in the evening and after noon, during about one hour or more. During these attacks, I felt in me all the wrath and furore of hell. I could allow no one to speak of Our Lord and Mother, and I could not bear seeing Their images, on which I spat and trod on under my feet [...] After the influence of the devil had passed and I remembered what I had done and said, I felt the most terrifying scruples; I thought I was the greatest criminal. I spent months of painful martyrdom. I would have much more to say on this matter, but I can't. My soul doesn't resist remembrance of such sufferings. [...]
>
> 13 June 1946
>
> My life is death; I still live the life of the dead. What an immense tomb it is, the vastness of the rottenness I am buried in; it causes me nausea, it causes me horror. I feel myself being eaten away by the worms hidden in this rottenness; I feel them moving and twisting in this putridity. And I have no other life than this or any other light than the blackness of my spirit. This sad blindness, that which doesn't allow me to see beyond these filthy, rotten, horrors.[23]

Alexandrina's narrative owes its existence to the injunction of her spiritual director, the Jesuit Father Mariano Pinho. Chronological narrative provides for an internal ordering of the otherwise chaotic material of her spiritual chaos into stages, from its origins to redemption, signs of redemption being periodically inserted into the narrative of crisis. Indeed, while remaining close to self-abjection, such sufferings, experienced in a state of identification with

22 Burton, *Holy Tears, Holy Blood.*

23 My translation of an excerpt of the text 'Autobiografia', attributted to Alexandrina Maria da Costa (known as Alexandrina de Balasar), <http://alexandrinabalasar.free.fr/ autobiografia_2.htm>. On the fixation of this text and the methodology concerning the use of sources displayed on the Internet, see my article, Marques, 'De corpo e alma na margem', 151-154.

Jesus on the cross, invariably pointed towards atonement for human sins. The dispositive of vicarious suffering, by temporarily deflecting the moral pain she identifies with – the moral pain that she *is* – towards an expiatory lamb identified with another – Christ and his religious symbol, the Eucharist – brings about a systole/diastole dynamic in which deflected suffering redeems, temporarily, the suffering with which she identifies:

> I feel Jesus crucified over all of my body; always His wounds on my hands, feet and heart, always his wounded body and the head surrounded by thorns. It isn't me, it is Jesus that is in me like this, it is Him that thus suffers; it is his Divine Heart that has thorns, a spear, swords, daggers and arrows. It is Him who suffers with Mother, and they both come to suffer in me. […].[24]

It is clear in these passages how the concept of 'sufferings' not only names, but actually builds the sense of Alexandrina's experience. For all the sheer physicality of her pain, Alexandrina understands and conveys her experience, not as illness, but as a suffering that 'makes sense' and is of worth to others.

Creating a medical niche for victim souls

The psychiatric critique eventually made the female sainthood model of mystical suffering harder to obtain than in previous centuries.[25] Alexandrina's case, for all its pre-modern facets, already testifies to this historical transformation, since the case was far from consensual even among the clergy of the time.

Biographies of Alexandrina intersperse accounts of her mystical experiences and mortifications with the numerous clinical examinations to which she was subject. These examinations, sometimes accompanied by difficult and long journeys, acquired the status of biographical events. Taking on the meaning of proof whether of a physical, moral or religious nature, overcome through faith and divine intercession, they prove crucial to the structure of her 'autobiography'. Many physicians are mentioned in such texts, invariably distinguished between those for and those against Alexandrina's sainthood. One particular doctor, Manuel Augusto Dias de Azevedo, is accorded a providential status, acting simultaneously as her bedside care provider, her confident and her mediator in his transcriptions of the messages issued whilst in 'ecstasy'. From the 1940s onwards, this devout physician became one of the main instigators of the cult of Alexandrina.

24 'Sentimentos da alma' (24 October 1947), <http://alex-balasar.blogspot.com/2011/11/eu-sou-sempre-mesma. html>.

25 On this model, see Albert, *Le sang et le ciel*.

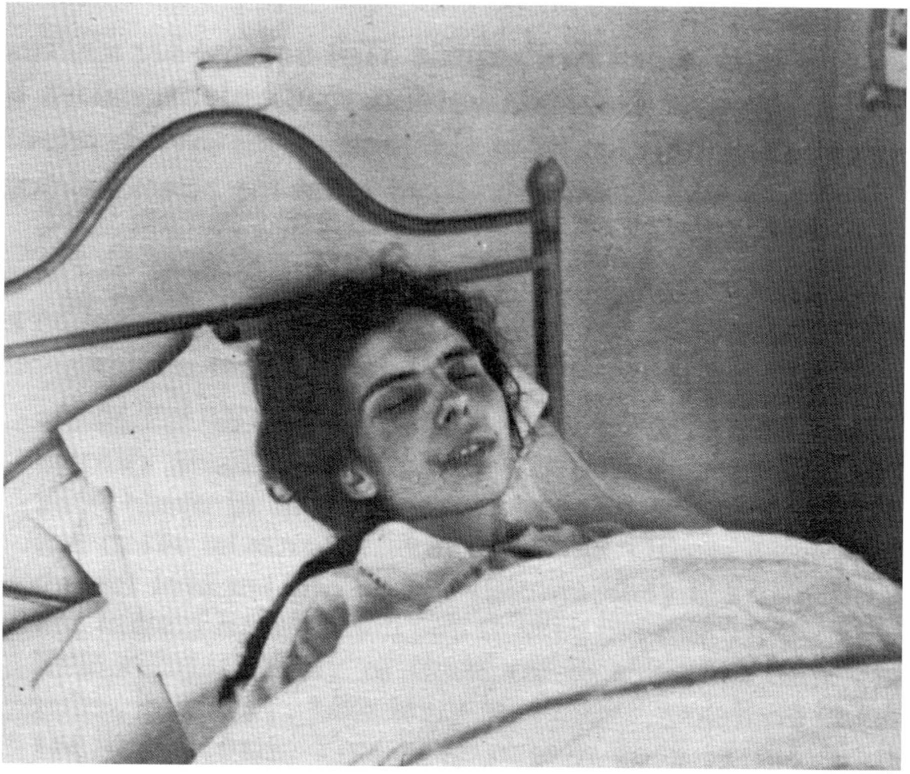

Alexandrina in ecstasy. This picture was taken in 1937 when Alexandrina was thirty-three years old.
[*Francis Johnston,* Alexandrina: The Agony and The Glor, *46*]

This doctor entered the scene after a previous attempt, by Alexandrina's spiritual director, to co-opt a Catholic physician favourable to a mystical interpretation of the phenomena. Indeed, in 1938, when Alexandrina began to relive the passion of Christ every Friday, Father Pinho fetched Catholic doctors to help discern the nature of what was happening with his penitent. The priest first called a Catholic professor of neurology and psychiatry and a clinical luminary of his time, Elísio de Moura, who examined Alexandrina. According to the Jesuit, Moura's examination dismissed any diagnosis of 'hysteria', which Pinho himself appears to have considered plausible. However, the psychiatrist stated that the case amounted to 'fraud and self-suggestion'. The Jesuit concluded that Elísio de Moura, who acknowledged not believing in either the phenomena of levitation or stigmatization, did not understand theology and mysticism.[26]

Three years later, Father Pinho found a doctor, a former seminarian, who also had a background in theology and was interested in mysticism, Dias de Azevedo. After observing the patient, the doctor delivered a clinical, theo-

26 Pinho, <alexandrinabalasar.free.fr/no_calvario_23.htm>.

logical and psychological diagnosis in a single stroke: from a clinical point of view, Alexandrina had transverse myelitis (an inflammation of the spinal cord); from a theological and mystical point of view, one could speak of a 'wonderful event'; and from a psychological point of view, Alexandrina was an intelligent and well balanced woman. He added that 'nothing, absolutely nothing, neither from the clinical nor the theological point of view, allowed for the classification of the phenomena observed as diabolic or natural'.[27] This left only a third etiological possibility: the ecstasies had a divine origin.

In the same year 1941, the Jesuit José Alves Terças authored the first known text on the 'ecstasies of Alexandrina', comparing these to the ecstasies of Anne Catherine Emmerich.[28] The article sparked a heated controversy among the Jesuits, eventually leading to the enforced exile of Father Pinho to Brazil. The prestigious Jesuit scientific journal *Brotéria* published an article by Agostinho Veloso, a Jesuit who presented himself as a Doctor in Ascetics and Mysticism of the University of Salamanca, countering such mystical interpretations. Entitled 'Mysticism and Medicine', this article illustrates the reluctance of the Church to attribute a supernatural character to phenomena susceptible to medical explanation. Even in cases of confirmed sainthood, the priest argued, one could observe the coexistence of supernatural and pathological phenomena. Excited by contact with God, the person's imagination remained naturally active once all supernatural action had come to an end. The author relied on the authority of Saint Thomas Aquinas and Bergson and illustrated the coexistence of mystical and pathological incidents with the case of Gemma Galgani, a young Italian mystic who died in 1903 and was canonized in 1940. The author did not explicitly mention Alexandrina of Balasar, but a note from the journal's director alluded to the case of 'a patient in Northern Portugal' as an example of the 'dangerous expansion' of visionary minds troubled by the supernatural.[29]

In 1943, Alexandrina stopped eating and drinking, ingesting only the sacred host in her daily communion. Following these events, the Archbishop of Braga, sceptical of the case, appointed a second commission of theologians to analyse Alexandrina. At the same time, the prelate urged Dias de Azevedo to keep his patient in isolation so that medical staff could observe her fully. Between 10 June and 20 July 1943, Alexandrina was observed in a hospital in the Porto region under the supervision of its director, the renowned neurologist Henrique Gomes de Araújo. Internment was subject to the acceptance of two conditions imposed by Azevedo: first, the team of doctors, who were primarily interested in her fasting, should also make a pronouncement on her mental faculties stating whether or not they were normal; secondly, the patient

27 Azevedo, <alexandrinabalasar.free.fr/no_calvario_23.htm>.
28 Terças, 'A martirizada do Calvário'.
29 Veloso, 'A Mística e a Medicina'.

should not be obliged to eat nor forced to take any drug by injection except in case of her express wish. With any possible therapeutic dimension thus curtailed, for doctors this internment constituted a clinical observation and a medical trial. However, to the supporters of Alexandrina's sainthood, this represented a method for obtaining medical certification on her fasting and psychical normality, and therefore an important element in the construction of a hagiographic narrative.[30]

The validity of the internment process and the resulting medical reports were at the mercy of various intrigues undertaken either by the doctors, priests or devotees. We should mention two medical reports, particularly significant on account of their inclusion in Alexandrina's hagiographical memory. One of them, signed by Gomes de Araújo, reads:

> At first glance, her aspect is perfect; and intellectually, emotionally and as far as her will is concerned she is normal; however, quickly she betrays being a carrier of fixed ideas, in a stereotyped and systematized form, living and feeling intensely and sincerely, without a shadow of mystification or fraud, the ideas that determine her abstinence. With regard to her physiognomic and moral features: lively expression, perfect, sweet, kind, caressing; sincere, unpretentious and fluid attitude. Neither exoticism nor sentimentality; neither shyness nor exalted voice. Natural conversation, intelligent and subtle.[31]

In this report, the doctor conveyed some details from the observation itself. To ensure control over what the patient ingested, he formed a monitoring team consisting of women who knew nothing of the specifics of Alexandrina. As a measuring device, a waterproof bag containing a salt solution was placed in the epigastrium region. Presumably, this instrument allowed to register variations in the content of Alexandrina's stomach, thus guaranteeing that no solids or liquids were ingested. The observation lasted forty days.

The report further stated that the surveillance was fully accomplished and that he could thus guarantee that the patient had not eaten, drunk, urinated or defecated during that time. Citing Charcot, he observed that the lack of appetite, defined as 'mental anorexia', actually constituted one of the most serious consequences of hysteria, to which he added: 'It is in part the case of Alexandrina. But only in part, since in this case total abstinence is accompanied by an interruption in the excretory function of the kidneys; in other words, no urination, no defecations.'[32] And the report concluded by stating

30 These events are described in several hagiographies of Alexandrina, including her 'Autobiography', <http://alexandrinabalasar.free.fr/ autobiografia>.

31 Araújo, *Relatório médico*, quoted in: <jejumalexandrina.blogspot.com>.

32 Ibid.

that she was a 'neurotic' whose pathological symptoms medicine could explain. However, medical advancements had to be made in order to explain abstinence from liquids and anuria.

The second report was signed by Alexandrina's assistant physician, Dias de Azevedo, and another doctor accompanying the observation, a psychiatry professor at the University of Oporto. Taking the form of a medical certificate, this report confirmed the fasting and anuria during internment and emphasized the extraordinary nature of such phenomena. It also certified the good mental faculties of the mystic and concluded by referring the phenomena observed every Friday to the territory of mysticism.[33] For Azevedo, who left unmentioned all the allusions to neurosis and 'fixed ideas', the report thus met the intended function of the internment: the fasting was real and Alexandrina was mentally normal.

However, in 1944, the commission of theologians published its own report, stating that the case of Alexandrina contained nothing of the supernatural and suggesting mental illness as an explanation. This document imposed silence on the clergy involved in the case and ordered the village priest to ensure the tranquillity of the 'sick woman'. In answer, supporters of the supernatural character of the phenomena argued that the disbelief of the commission of theologians, and specifically its chairman, another Jesuit priest, derived directly from the scepticism then prevailing at Rome's Gregorian University. Such scepticism could be traced back to its roots and was first caused by the reception of the case of Therese Neumann (1898-1962) by the studies of Agostino Gemelli, a renowned biologist and Franciscan priest (founder of Milan's Catholic University), and of a Polish Jesuit teacher of psychology, Paul Siwek.[34]

While Gemelli attained notoriety in the scientific milieus for articulating biological and medical sciences within the ontological and epistemological framework of neo-Thomism, Siwek seems to have been highly influential in reframing the Catholic understanding of mysticism in a period witnessing advances in materialist science. A professor at the Gregorian University between 1921 and 1930, Siwek, an eminent specialist on Aristotle, devoted much energy to refuting Espinosa and the theory of metempsychosis, which he held as present in Buddhism and spiritualism. Additionally, he also entrusted the natural sciences with the mission of bringing non-believers from the intellectual territories of individualism, materialism and Freudianism to the Catholic faith. Translated into several languages, including Portuguese, Siwek was indeed the author of a reference work on Therese Neumann, *The Riddle of*

33 Azevedo and Lima, *Relatório médico*, <http://jejumalexandrina.blogspot.com/2009/11/jj5.html>.

34 Azevedo quoted in: <http://alexandrina.balasar.free.fr/doutor_azevedo_e_alexandrina.htm>.

Konnersreuth. A Psychological and Religious Study of Theresa Neumann (1953) and produced the psychology textbook officially adopted at the Gregorian University and other Catholic universities (*Psychologia Metaphysica*, first edition 1939).[35]

The controversy continued especially in 1947 following a new article by the Jesuit Agostinho Veloso in *Brotéria*, that now explicitly mentioned Alexandrina, to whom the author applied the notion of a 'psychosis of wonders'.[36] With the clergy now more discreet about the case, the response in support of Alexandrina's mysticism again came from the medical domain, with the assistant doctor questioning the authority of the Jesuit in matters of psychiatry.[37] The partisans of mystical interpretations also mobilized philosophical authorities, Bergson first and foremost, and international medical authorities, in particular the French Catholic doctors Antoine Imbert-Gourbeyre (1818-1912) and Henri Bon (1885-1958), both authors of books on miraculous cures.[38]

This case thus shows the inversion of hitherto traditional positions: while medical authority supported the religious nature of the observed phenomenon, religious authorities, relying on psychiatric terms, argued for its pathological character. Together with the analysis on Fátima above, this suggests that the Catholic Church had displaced the possibility of religious wonders from the terrain of corporeal mysticism to that of Marian apparitions. In this process, science, and psychiatry in particular, played a major role in shaping new configurations, including identifiable scientific arguments, procedures and authorities.

The religious incorporation of a medical experiment

Besides these religious and theological shifts, the clinical experiment on Alexandrina is significant in terms of the changes in the context and content of psychiatry. Between the 1920s and the 1940s, a process of institutionalization and the de-politicizing of psychiatry took place. The first stage in the consolidation of psychiatry as an autonomous clinical field relied heavily on the action of militant Republican psychiatrists and, from 1910 onwards, on the proximity of the leading psychiatrists to the political powers. Motivated by their political campaign against the social power of priests, psychiatrists employed the concepts of hysteria and delusion prolifically as a means of attacking religious beliefs and Catholic models of sainthood.[39]

35 See biographical note in: <www.catholicauthors.com/siwek.html>.
36 Veloso, 'Mística e jornalismo', 5.
37 <http://alexandrinabalasar.free.fr/alex_veloso_2.htm>.
38 Azevedo, article dated 31 August 1953, <http://alexandrina.balasar.free.fr/doutor_azevedo_e_alexandrina.htm>.
39 Marques, 'Uma frágil camada de Razão', 198-209.

After World War I, however, the struggles between Republicans and the Catholic Church became appeased. Simultaneously, new ideas entered the landscape of psychiatry, clearly in opposition to the concept of 'hysteria' as it had been developed by Charcot. Two of the doctors examining Alexandrina played important roles in this psychiatric renewal. The neurologist Gomes de Araújo pioneered criticism of hysteria in his doctoral thesis through the concept of 'pithiatisme', coined by Joseph Babinski (1857-1932) in France.[40] Furthermore, Elísio de Moura – the abovementioned doctor who observed Alexandrina in the late 1930s – echoed the idea that 'hysteria' was too broad a concept to be employed accurately in clinical reasoning. Following the approaches of Babinski and Araújo, Moura replaced in the very first work on anorexia published in Portugal (1947) 'hysteria' with 'pithiatisme', which referred exclusively to 'functional troubles' susceptible to reproduction through controlled experiments and extinguishable by means of an 'external influence'.[41] Thus reformulated, the concept of 'hysteria' was meant to exclude phenomena such as 'prophetic dreams', 'demonomania' (delusions of being possessed) and stigmatization from its extent.[42] Simultaneously, Moura introduced the notion of 'mental anorexia' as distinct from the older notions of 'nervous anorexia', coined by the British physician William Gull (1816-1890), and 'hysterical anorexia', developed by the French specialist Ernest-Charles Lasègue (1816-1883), which were both articulated within the frame of hysteria.[43]

Far from being an archaism or the result of scientific ignorance, the experiment with Alexandrina belongs entirely to this new context. Although incorporating some local specificities linked to its religious framing, her analysis resonated transnational psychiatric developments, which were not alien to the comparable cases of Gemma Galgani, Marthe Robin and Therese Neumann. Thus, Alexandrina's case may be historically situated at a specific point on the intersection of religious and scientific mutations.

The medical tribulations to which Alexandrina was subject, became a crucial factor in the construction of her religious persona. In her *Autobiography*, the observations carried out by Elísio de Moura are portrayed as a form of torture and humiliation. In addition, this text includes her ordeal at the hospital in Oporto designed to have her mystical phenomena observed by doctors. The trip to the hospital is described as an adventurous and painful Golgotha. Entering the hospital, her body and face were covered, as if she was dead ('It seemed I was in a coffin'). The text does not obscure the resulting clinical diagnosis classifying Alexandrina as 'hysterical' with a 'religious delusion'. Nevertheless, the diagnosis emphasizes that she did not eat anything other than the

40 Aráujo, *Histeria, pithiatismo.*
41 Moura, *Anorexia mental*, 102.
42 Ibid., 103.
43 Brumberg, *Fasting Girls*, 117-118 and 125-132.

consecrated wafer and neither urinated nor defecated throughout her hospital stay. Once again, the internment, extended from the originally planned thirty days to forty, took on a religious significance: just like Jesus in the desert, she had her forty days and forty nights of temptation and fasting. After the successful clinical trial, Alexandrina describes her reconciliation with the medical team and the great public recognition expressed in 'showers of flowers' and perfumes thrown by the devotees. In sum, her contacts with the medical world had become tightly interwoven into her religious experience. Eventually, the supporters of Alexandrina's sainthood hailed the clinical report as proof of the reality of her mystical phenomena.[44]

Conclusion: belief processes and embodied epistemologies

By way of conclusion, I would like to briefly consider the notion of embodied epistemologies, as elaborated in medical and religious anthropology in the last few decades. An article published by Margaret Lock in 1993 constitutes a fine approach to this concept. Lock offers indeed a concise analysis of the theoretical frames intent on overcoming 'a radical separation of knowledge and practice [...] through decentering the cognitive construction of knowledge', in order to illuminate the ways in which conditions and processes of knowledge inform bodily experience.[45] More recently, this line of inquiry has been developed through more specific concepts such as 'somatic modes of attention' (Csordas), 'strategic suffering' (Hunt), as a means of linking experience and illness-and-healing narratives.[46] In a similar vein, David Morgan argues that the acts of seeing supernatural beings must be understood within historical 'regimes of embodiment'.[47] These concepts further develop the idea that corporeal experiences are informed by, and act upon, collective frames of cognition. This is the case for Fátima's visions and Alexandrina's suffering, as the above analysis shows that the experiences of these religious mediators reflected different epistemological configurations and related belief processes. Alexandrina's case is particularly illuminating: disputes around hysteria held a significant impact on the process through which her religious persona took shape. Indeed, conducted within the psychiatric context of the debate on pithiatisme and related notions of anorexia, the experiment was crucial to detach the fasting from the ensemble of symptoms and to assert its corporeal reality, and thus the reality of the Catholic concept of miraculous inedia. This resonated not only in the scientific milieu, but also in the course of Alexandrina's

44 Alexandrina Costa, *Autobiografia*, <http://alexandrinabalasar.free.fr/ autobiografia_2.htm>.

45 Lock, 'Cultivating the Body', 136.

46 Csordas, *Body/ Meaning/ Healing*, 136-137, 258-259; Hunt, 'Strategic Suffering'.

47 Morgan, *The Embodied Eye*, 51.

mystical life, with the fasting dethroning the ecstasies as the chief signal of mystical authenticity.

While more obvious in Alexandrina's story, a perspective on experience as embodied epistemology helps to us to systematically compare the two cases along the lines of (1) objects of belief, (2) subject and credibility, and (3) the reported communications between earthly life and the beyond.

1) In Marian apparitions, bodies presented as objects of belief are otherworldly. Therefore, science cannot be mobilized directly in their construction. The process by means of which these bodies become believable interacts with the formalization of images representing the apparition, is a process some scholars have analysed as a dialectics of interface and iconicity, or recognition and iconization.[48] In Fatima's case, Church authorities played a crucial role in the initial stage leading to the discursive stabilization of the image, allowing the identification of the apparition with the Virgin Mary. In contrast, in the victim soul case, the body supporting belief in miraculous phenomena was this-worldly and simultaneously exceptional. Thus, while also reflecting a religious model – the Catholic tradition of mystical women – its material corporeality made it an object of scientific observation.

2) Again, as far as the subjective validity of the experience is concerned, the two cases show a few differences. In Marian apparitions, psychiatric arguments referring to the seers surface in the apologetic reports as a means of reinforcing their credibility. Yet, similarly to other apparitions, and in the logic of Catholic miracle validation as codified by Pope Benedict XIV (1740-1758), they were instrumental in eliminating obstacles to belief.[49] Instead, the credibility of the victim soul was tightly linked to psychiatric arguments, mobilized by both supporters and opponents of religious interpretations.

3) Marian apparitions and victim souls converge in the idea that the communication between the immanent and transcendent planes is observed in the suspension of the laws of nature. However, in the former case, such suspension is occasional and limited to the sacred site, whilst in the latter the natural order is continuously challenged. In Fátima, the scientific worldview is crucial in creating the space in which transcendence is manifested: the 'miracle of the sun' is a breach in the laws of nature, just as much as miraculous cures are a breach in biological processes. Similarly, the soul victim Alexandrina asserts the truthfulness of her experience by stating exception to nature. Yet, inedia and repeated ecstasies render its exceptionality a long-term condition.

48 Ibid., 89-92; Scheer, 'What She Looks Like', 442-467.

49 Jansen and Notermans, 'From Vision to Cult Site', 83, 85; Chiron, *Enquête sur les apparitions de la Vierge*, 44.

Alexandrina thus embodied a state of exception to nature in which the earthly and divine orders communicated.[50]

This scheme is tentative and overlooks a few common and different features. For instance, site and public played different roles in the two cases, as the sacred and public site of the apparitions contrasts with the profane, yet private, site of the victim soul phenomena (the household and hospital bedrooms). Some common aspects may also be referred to, in particular the importance of the theme of expiatory suffering. Still, this comparison allows us to emphasize the notion that the modernizing world of miraculous Catholicism integrated scientific dimensions either as an argument for the realness of supernatural or mystical phenomena (mostly in the case of Marian apparitions) or as a competing interpretative frame to combat, negotiate with and virtually co-opt (in the case of victim souls). Nonetheless, the cognitive and experiential frames typical of modernity appear to have favoured Marian apparitions to the detriment of victim soul mysticism. Even in the world of folk Catholicism, populated by mediating figures such as fasting girls and the Virgin, Alexandrina's ever agonizing and self-effacing body was at odds with the glorious body of the Lady of Fatima, of incomparable beauty and brilliance, and, above all else, left unscathed by science and theology.

50 In this line of thinking, anthropologist João Pina Cabral referred to Alexandrina and other similar cases in the region through the lenses of liminality, as analysed by A. Van Gennep and Victor Turner. See Cabral, *Sons of Adam, Daughters of Eve*, 218-224.

A QUESTION OF COMPETENCE AND AUTHORITY

LAY VIEWS ON THE MEDICAL EXAMINATIONS OF THE MARIAN APPARITION SERIES IN 1930S BELGIUM

TINE VAN OSSELAER*

In August 1934, the Belgian author Louis Wilmet complained about the medical examiners responsible for the investigation of a series of apparitions in Belgium. In his opinion, their goals and the perspective they had adopted hindered communication with them, even making this impossible.[1] Notwithstanding his remarks, Wilmet, like so many other interested observers of the series of apparitions, had initially been keen to have the doctors involved. In line with the Catholic Church's stance, he believed that a medical examination of the exceptional phenomena was required before they could be accepted as 'real' (the 'medicalization' of the miracle).[2] Wilmet and others thereby intended to put the interest in the apparition series shown by the doctors to tactical use in promotional campaigns, and by citing them as authorities, aimed to convince others of their own beliefs.[3] In this article, I want to address this inconsistency in their relationship to medicine and examine the ways in which the lay voices involved alternated between demanding and

* Research supported by the Research Foundation Flanders.

1 Archives of the Diocese of Namur (ADN), L.42. 1. Louis Wilmet: Louis Wilmet to Princess de Croÿ, 14 August 1934: 'Je crois pouvoir conclure que toutes ces enquêtes sont rien moins que sérieuses et que les enquêteurs et les autorités ne parlent pas le même langage que nous...'

2 Szabo, 'Seeing is Believing?', 211; Desmazières, 'Psychology against Medicine?', 1192: 'the medical intrusion in a field traditionally controlled by theology'.

3 On 'citation' as a tactic to promote belief or mistrust, see De Certeau, *The Practice of Everyday Life*, 188.

criticizing the medical examinations of the series of phenomena that puzzled Belgium in the 1930s.[4]

Research on the involvement of doctors at apparition sites has primarily focused on Lourdes and the *miraculés*. Scholars such as Ruth Harris, Jason Szabo, Suzanne Kaufman and Andreas Kotulla have demonstrated how the sanctuary became the centre of French discussions over faith and science.[5] It would be wrong, however, to describe the Lourdes case solely in terms of an opposition of faith and science. By the 1870s, interest in the medical substantiation of miraculous cures had increased and the *miraculés* were requested to send in medical certificates when pleading their cause.[6] Furthermore, by creating the Bureau of Medical Verifications (Bureau des Constations Médicales) in 1883, the Church accepted the need for scientific verification and the value of the epistemological criteria of modern medicine (which would strengthen rather than weaken belief in miracles).[7] Moreover, while opponents of Lourdes commented upon the reliability and objectivity of the observations, the hygienic circumstances and mass hysteria, they were also impressed by the therapeutic results obtained at the site. They no longer saw the cures as fraud, but now looked for explanations and discussed the miraculous cures in debates on faith healing, hypnotism, physiological magnetism[8] and hydrotherapy.[9] Furthermore, while they might not have agreed on the explanations for the cures, anticlerics and their religious opponents did have some features in common. Their practice of the 'public display of patients' was one of them. While Charcot and his Salpêtrière colleagues observed patients' bodies during public lessons, Dr Boissarie, the head of the Bureau, exhibited them to a Parisian public in an attempt to convince them of the permanence of the miraculous cure.[10] Catholic references to the body as 'proof' can also be noted in

4 'Medical' refers here to both a psychological interpretation and a medical approach: both were described as 'medical' in the sources.

5 According to Ruth Harris, Lourdes reasserted 'the importance and even the existence of the miraculous at precisely the moment when science attained an apparently unquestionable authority'. Harris, *Lourdes*, 289.

6 Ibid., 302.

7 Ibid., 307. See also Szabo, 'Seeing is Believing?', 212, where it is argued that they wanted to 'generate observations – clinical facts – convincing enough to silence the critics of Lourdes'.

8 Harris, *Lourdes*, 320, 351, 353; in particular see 355: 'In an age of anti-clericalism, when science and religion were deemed antithetical to one another, Lourdes generated an unusual relationship between them. Both gave some ground, and neither remained untouched by the other'. See also Harris, 'Les miraculés de Lourdes', 295; and Kotulla, *Nach Lourdes*, 116.

9 Kotulla, *Nach Lourdes*, 115.

10 Comparing pictorial sources, Harris notes how an 1887 rendering of one such lesson depicts the 'coldness of scientific rationalism', while a more humane and sympathetic treatment of the patients is to be observed in the pictures of the questioning by the Bureau in 1880 and 1900. Harris, *Lourdes*, 329.

the images of the *miraculés* on numerous postcards,[11] or in the public display of bronze replicas of the bones of the *miraculé* Pierre De Rudder in the Lourdes museum.[12]

While Pierre's bones were marvelled at by the 'common' layperson and the images of the *miraculés* were collected by pilgrims of all kinds, the discussions over science and religion were most often between experts. Nevertheless, some scholars have hinted at a lay response to this medical involvement in Lourdes. According to Andreas Kotulla, the activities of the Bureau created, at least in the Catholic lay public, 'eine wissenschaftlich-medizini-sche Glaubwürdigkeit'.[13] Ruth Harris, however, has a more negative view of the Catholic lay response. In her opinion, Catholic scepticism concerning the doctors' findings continued, and there remained a rather negative attitude towards the 'medical inadequacy and even torture at the hands of science'. She adds:

> ... while the Church increasingly depended on medical opinion, the perception of the faithful remained tied to popular traditions generally heedless of doctors. This tension was never resolved, and many cured individuals simply refused to undergo the grueling process of medical investigation and the subsequent episcopal investigation, preferring instead their subjective certainty and the empirical verification of families and local communities.[14]

The Lourdes case and its reception is by far one of the best studied, but interest in twentieth-century apparitions is also slowly increasing. Interestingly, research on these modern cases centres on the medical investigations of the visionaries. For example, in her work on the German sites of Heede and Heroldsbach, Anna Maria Zumholz indicates how, in the nineteenth and twentieth centuries, various disciplines in the expanding field of psychology offered explanations for what once had been deemed inexplicable phenomena,

11 Suzanne Kaufman describes this public display of the bodies at meetings as part of what she calls 'scientific sensationalism'. This sensationalism can also be traced in the medically substantiated narratives about miraculous cures (spread via the Bureau, among others) or in the images of the *miraculés*. See Kaufman, *Consuming Visions*, 96-97. According to Jason Szabo, in this use of photo iconography, the supporters of Lourdes followed in the footsteps of Charcot and thereby created a 'new group of medico-religious artefacts'. Szabo, 'Seeing is Believing?', 217.

12 Only a small scar remained, pointing to the fracture that had been thought incurable and offering 'physical proof' of the miraculous cure. Harris, *Lourdes*, 344.

13 Kotulla, *Nach Lourdes*, 114.

14 Harris, *Lourdes*, 309 and 307; in particular see 355: 'For by continuing to limit the domain of the supernatural, science had the effect of undermining the judgements of Catholic believers. The subjective assessments of pilgrims, as well as the empirical evaluations of relatives, neighbours and friends, became of less value than those of medical experts.'

describing these as hallucinations, eidetic phenomena, hypnotic trance and hysteria.[15]

This growing interest in psychological explanations has also been pointed to in work on the Belgian wave of apparitions.[16] Agnès Desmazières has described the Beauraing case (the first of the Belgian apparition series) as exemplary of 'the clash between the emerging psychological interpretation of apparitions and the medical approach which has prevailed since Lourdes'.[17] She notes how – since the visionaries refused to undergo physiological tests while they were in ecstasy – the attention shifted towards the questioning of the visionaries after the apparitions, paving the path for psychologists.[18] While I will also discuss the medical interest in the Beauraing apparitions, my focus here will not be limited to the Walloon site. By examining the medical involvement at the various Belgian sites, I will also include places where the physical 'proof' (derived from the visionaries' bodies) remained important. Moreover, I will also consider the miraculous cures. In addition to broadening the study to the whole Belgian series of apparitions and to the two types of bodies under scrutiny (those of the visionaries and those of the *miraculés*), I have also changed reception levels. My focus is on the lay reception of the doctors' activities, which seems to have been more complex than the mere rejection found in the case of Lourdes.

The Belgian series of apparitions and the doctors involved

To be more precise, the discussion with which we are concerned took place over a series of Marian apparitions that swept across Belgium from November 1932 until around 1935. Apparitions and paramystical events, such as stigmata, bleeding crucifixes and miracles of the sun, were reported at approximately 40 sites, with hundreds of visionaries involved. In line with the 'modern' apparition-type occurring at Lourdes, the apparitions were public and serial. People knew when to visit these sites and did so in large numbers.

15 Zumholz, 'Die Resistenz des katholischen Milieus'. In her more elaborate analysis of the Heede case, she points out how the discussions were primarily between the public authorities (later the Gestapo) and the medical experts. The psychological health of the girl visionaries from Heede was tested, including their eidetic capacities and their susceptibility to suggestion. See Zumholz, *Volksfrömmigkeit*, 348.

16 For other, brief, overviews of the doctors' involvement during the Belgian 1930s series of apparitions, see 'The arrogance of the doctors' 'Arrogance des médecins' in Joset, *Dossiers de Beauraing*, 160-210. Together with Mgr Toussaint, Joset also included a brief note in *Beauraing*, 98-100. See also the references in biographies, for example, on the work of Prof. De Greeff in Casselman, *Etienne De Greeff*, 70-78.

17 Desmazières, 'Psychology against Medicine?', 1193. For this psychological interest in Beauraing, see also Bossant, *Het dossier van de verschijningen te Beauraing*.

18 Desmazières, 'Psychology against Medicine?', 1201.

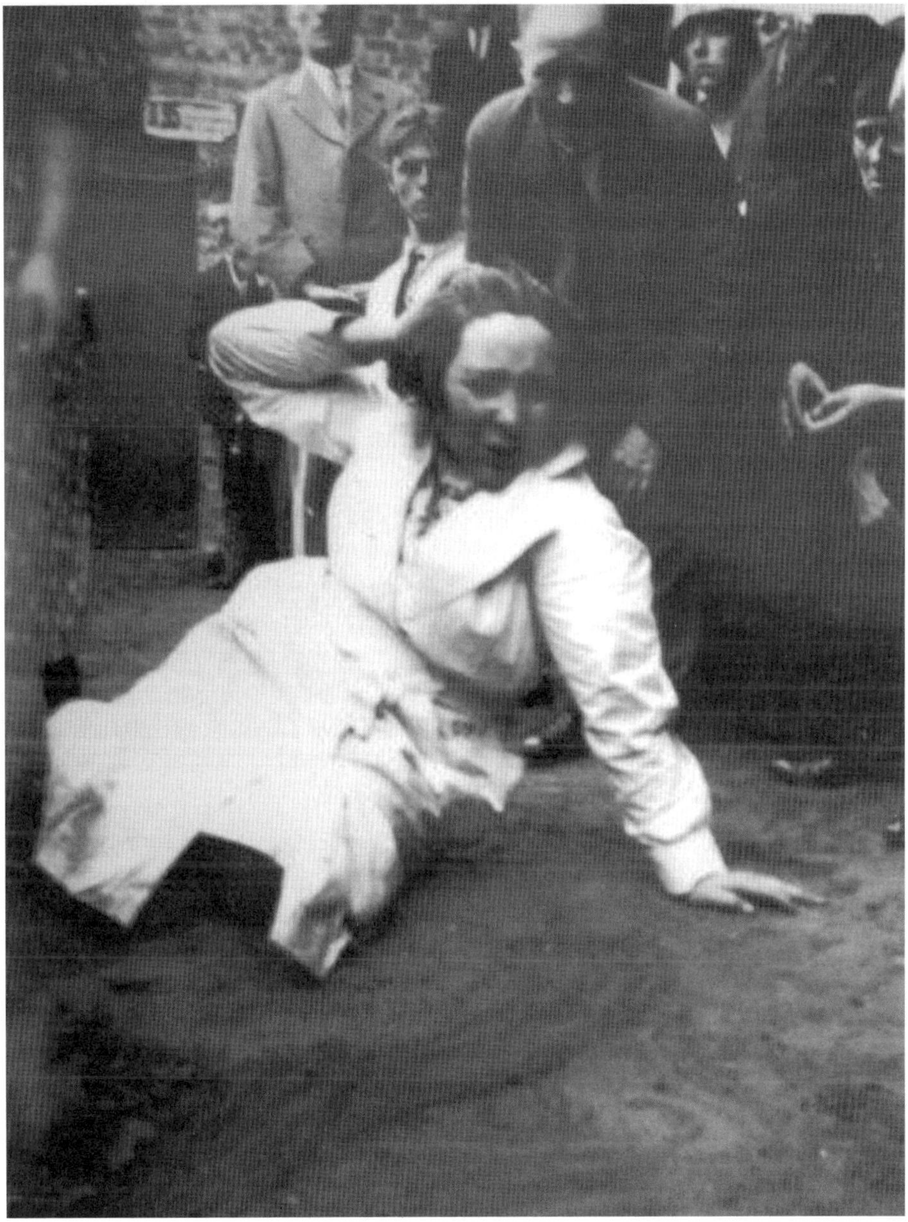

Elisabeth Cornelis, visionary of the Lokeren apparition series (summer 1934).
[*Ghent, Archives of the Diocese of Ghent, Onkerzele*]

Among them were numerous doctors driven by professional curiosity, eager to see the phenomena with their own eyes, and – if possible – run some tests and participate in the questioning of the visionaries. Their presence at the sites did not go unnoticed and was frequently commented upon by the lay witnesses.[19] The interest of the Belgian doctors was similar to that of their colleagues at other European sites.[20] Thanks to these precedents – referred to in Catholic periodicals (e.g. about miraculous cures in Oostakker) and witnessed on pilgrimages – the doctors were accepted as necessary at the Belgian sites, as 'authorities' who had to be involved. However, their competence-based 'authority' was quite different from that of the Catholic Church and, *in casu*, the bishops.[21] As we shall see, this difference was reflected in the attitudes of the laypeople.

From the first attestations in Beauraing onwards, doctors found their way to the apparition sites. Initially, only Dr Goethals (from Hastière-par-delà) and the local Dr Maistriaux were present at the Walloon site.[22] However, the number of doctors soon increased and in January 1933 the police had to limit the numbers entering the garden where the Beauraing apparitions could best be viewed. Permits to enter the site had been handed out too readily and the number of doctors already exceeded one hundred.[23] The doctors not only observed the apparitions in Beauraing, they also conducted experiments (on 8 December)[24] and participated in the questioning of child visionaries after their encounters with Mary.[25] Other apparition sites also caught the attention

19 I use the term 'lay' to refer to non-clerical witnesses of the series of apparitions; the clergy, of course, also commented on the events – but that is quite a different story.

20 Harris, *Lourdes*, 355; Szabo, 'Seeing is Believing?'; Duffin, *Medical Miracles*; Kaufman, *Consuming Visions*, 95-134; Harris, 'Les miraculées de Lourdes'. On the relationship between medicine and religion in discussing these phenomena in Belgium, see Velle, 'De geneeskunde', 1 and 13; Lachapelle, 'Between Miracle and Sickness', 88, footnote 21; Falleyn, *Hysterie*, 81 and 112.

21 On the difference between *auctoritas*/authority (counterpart: trust) and *potestas* (counterpart: obedience) see Krieger, 'The idea of Authority'.

22 On 6 December 1932 – in fact, too late to attend the apparitions. The local doctor of Beauraing wrote the first book on the Beauraing apparitions (*Que se passe-t-il à Beauraing?*) and a follow-up (*Les dernières apparitions de Beauraing*) at the request of Rex, the publishing house of the Catholic Action youth movement. Charlier, *Leon Degrelle*, 76.

23 Archives of the Sanctuary of Beauraing (ASB), Comité Pro Maria/Aurélien Pierroux, 1932-1933: Speech given in Brussels on 25 January 1933 by Louis Wilmet on Beauraing after La Salette, Lourdes, and Fatima.

24 After the children heard about the first experiments they complained. It was agreed upon that only six doctors (whom the children trusted) would be allowed to enter the apparition site during their visions. They were, however, not allowed to touch them. Joset, *Dossiers de Beauraing*, 170.

25 Archives of the Congregation for the Doctrine of the Faith (ACDF), Devotiones Variae (Dev. Var.), Beauraing, 1933.2 (794/1933), box 4: Session 10 (14 June 1935) of the Diocesan Commission of Namur. The names of the doctors present during questioning are listed in Joset, *Dossiers de Beauraing*, 162-168.

of doctors, most often that of the local doctors. While the tests and questioning at these other sites seem to have been more ad hoc,[26] in Beauraing they developed into well-organized events. It is most likely that those involved modelled their activities on what they knew about Lourdes: Dr Goethals, the first doctor who had shown an interest in the apparitions, participated in the *Pèlerinages Namurois* to Lourdes, and was highly familiar with its medical bureau and examinations.[27] Nevertheless, in spite of this more formal character, the Beauraing group of doctors, although tolerated and approved by the bishop of Namur, was never officially recognized by the bishops.

The doctors' involvement in the Belgian apparition series gained a more formal character with the creation of a medical commission on 2 December 1933.[28] The contemporaries seem to have been well aware of the official sanctioning, for when one of its members first went to the Flemish apparition site of Onkerzele on 8 December 1933, a lay commentator noted: 'it was thus the first time in the history of the apparitions in Belgium that an observation with an official character took place'.[29] The commission,[30] created in Brussels at the request of the archbishop and under the direction of the Medical Society of Saint Luc,[31] was charged with two tasks: its members were to examine (across the entire country): (1) the visionaries and (2) the miraculous healings that

26 See e.g. mention of the presence of doctors at the original Lokeren site, watching Gustave, s.n., 'De verschijningen te Lokeren', *Het Laatste Nieuws*, 16 November 1933, 2.

27 Joset, *Dossiers de Beauraing*, 161.

28 In relation to the decision process, there were four stages of examination of an apparition set out by Benedict XIV (1675-1758), see Chiron, *Enquête sur les apparitions de la Vierge*, 44: 1. The personality of the visionary; 2. The content of the apparition; 3. The nature and form of the apparition; and 4. The goal of the apparition. Apparitions must also pass a triple critique: 1. Historical judgement (critique of the testimonies); 2. Human judgement (psychological); 3. Theological scrutiny. A commission was made up of theologians, canonists, medics and – sometimes – other experts. As for the psychological investigation, as early as 1777, a text had been published on *Institutiones theologicae mysticae*, in which Dom Schram listed 19 signs which, when detected in a visionary, might render the apparitions suspect.

29 ADN, L.42, Wilmet III: Confidential note on the medical commission: 'C'est donc la première fois dans l'histoire des apparitions en Belgique qu'une observation à caractère officiel a eu lieu.'

30 It is not really clear on whose initiative the commission was established: there is a note on an episcopal gathering of 24-25 July 1933 indicating that a medical commission investigating Beauraing and Banneux would be established, consisting of members of the Medical Society of Saint Luc. See Archives of the Archdiocese of Mechelen (AAM): Reports of the meetings of the bishops, 24-25 July 1933, IX: *Les faits de Beauraing et Banneux*. There is also a letter from Dr Wibo, head of the Medical Society of Saint Luc, sent to Mgr Heylen on 22 September 1933, in which he remarks that it is absolutely necessary to examine the healings, just as this is done in Lourdes. ACDF, Dev. Var., Beauraing, 1933.2 (794/1933), 24: Letter from Cawet to his Excellence, in a report sent to Mgr Micara, nuncio in Brussels.

31 Velle, 'Het verenigingsleven', 105, after the First World War it was established in various cities. From 1923, it had its own periodical. In 1935, the Belgian movement had approximately 1,200 members.

were attested to at the various sites. The goal of the commission was to determine whether or not the phenomena could be explained in a natural way. If that was not the case, they would be subject to a theological examination.[32]

The commission was not made up of the local doctors who had been frequenting the sites. The task of examining the series of apparitions was now in the hands of academic scholars. Dr Fransen (professor of psychology at the University of Ghent) was in charge of the investigation of the Flemish sites; Dr Gailly (a psychiatrist from Charleroi) examined the Beauraing visionaries and visited Banneux; and Dr Paul Van Gehuchten (professor of neurology in the medical faculty at Leuven) investigated the miraculous cures.[33] The commission thus primarily consisted of scholars with an interest in psychology, bound to examine the two types of people involved: the visionaries and the *miraculés*. However, the scholars also received assistance from other doctors, and we find the names of their various assistants in the reports on their activities at the sites.[34] Moreover, since the commission was only installed in December 1933, one year after the apparition series had begun (when at least 20 sites had already been reported), its members also called upon the expertise of the doctors who had examined the phenomena at the sites before they did.[35]

The appointment of the commission members did not occur without discussion. It is important to note that even before they became officially involved, the members of this medical commission, Dr Van Gehuchten, Dr Fransen and Dr Gailly, had expressed their opinions on the series of apparitions. They were clearly interested in what was happening, and in the minds of some of their contemporaries they were already too 'involved' and prejudiced to be able to examine the wave of apparitions with open minds. Their statements at meetings of the Medical Society of Saint Luc[36] and articles published in its periodical, *Saint Luc Médical*,[37] and *Les Études Carmélitaines* created doubts in lay minds about their impartiality.

32 ADN, L.42, Wilmet IV: Answer from Lenain to Wilmet, 8 August 1934.
33 AAM, Processus circa assertas apparitions et revelations (Processus): Session 9 (12 November 1935) of the commission of Malines.
34 Parish Archive Onkerzele (PAO), 58, III. B., national 9: Stenographic report of the questioning, 21 January 1934.
35 For example, Prof. Fransen contacted Dr Verschueren about Onkerzele, AAM, Processus, B.XI.2. Documenta 'G IV': Letter from Van der Maeren to Mgr Coppieters, 16 April 1934.
36 ADN, L.42, Wilmet III: Letter from Lenain to Wilmet, s.d.
37 Issue 4 (1933): the issue also included articles by the doctors Goedseels, Maistriaux, De Greeff, Gailly and Fransen. The periodical published six issues a year – so most probably July, as, according to Casselman, *Etienne De Greeff*, 73, it was halfway through 1933.

Lay reception of the doctors' activities

For the laypeople present at the various sites, corporeal phenomena seemed to provide 'objective' proof of what was happening. Two types of bodies provided support for the claims of supernatural intervention: 1) the ecstatic bodies of the visionaries and 2) the miraculously cured bodies. Examining these was considered the task of the doctors, but their activities were closely scrutinized by laypeople.

Dangerous and/or necessary: the medical experiments

In various reports, the supporters of the apparitions commented on the impression the medical experiments left on the bystanders. These documents were probably sent from one supporter to another and none were ever made public. However, they document the care with which the experiments were observed and the results evaluated. We are particularly well informed about the activities of Dr Careels (from Lier) at the Onkerzele site. This was a major apparition site in Flanders that first drew attention in August 1933, when Leonie Van Dijck claimed to see the Virgin. Soon afterwards, a second series of apparitions began, involving several other visionaries. It is this series of apparitions that Dr Careels was studying in December 1933 and early 1934.

The reports all describe the external features of the experiments. They document how Careels felt the pulse of the visionaries during the apparitions, touched their eyeballs, stabbed their feet, burned matches underneath their hands and attempted to bend their fingers and hands. Most of these reports emphasized how these experiments did not trigger any reflex responses from the visionaries.[38] However, Louis Wilmet (never a supporter of the Flemish series of apparitions)[39] and A. Martin believed they had seen something quite different. A. Martin, for example, documented how one of the experiments by Dr Fransen managed to force the visionary, Berthonia, out of her ecstasy on 21 January 1934. The result of the experiment created further doubts about the 'authenticity' of this visionary, which had already been growing in his mind.[40]

38 AAM, Processus, B IX.A. 1 (19/10-28/12/1933): Report by Honoré Vermeire about Onkerzele, 8 December 1933; Ibid., B IX.A. 1. (19/10-28/12/1933): Report by Honoré Vermeire, 18 December 1933; Ibid., B IXa2 (6/1-31/3/1934): Report by Alfred Magain about 6 January 1934; Ibid., B IXa1: Report by Vermeire, 9 February 1934; Ibid., B IXa2 (6/1-31/3/1934): Report by Sebruyns-Desmet on 30 March 1934.

39 AAM, Processus, B IX.A. 1 (19/10-28/12/1933): Report by Wilmet on 28 December 1933: he reported that in Onkerzele, Dr Careels tested their insensitivity using a flame, that he was not really sure about the results, that Berthonia had moved a little and that it might have been the result of the flame.

40 AAM, Processus, B IXa2 (6/1-31/3/1934): Letter from A. Martin to the secretary of the bishop of Ghent, 31 January 1934.

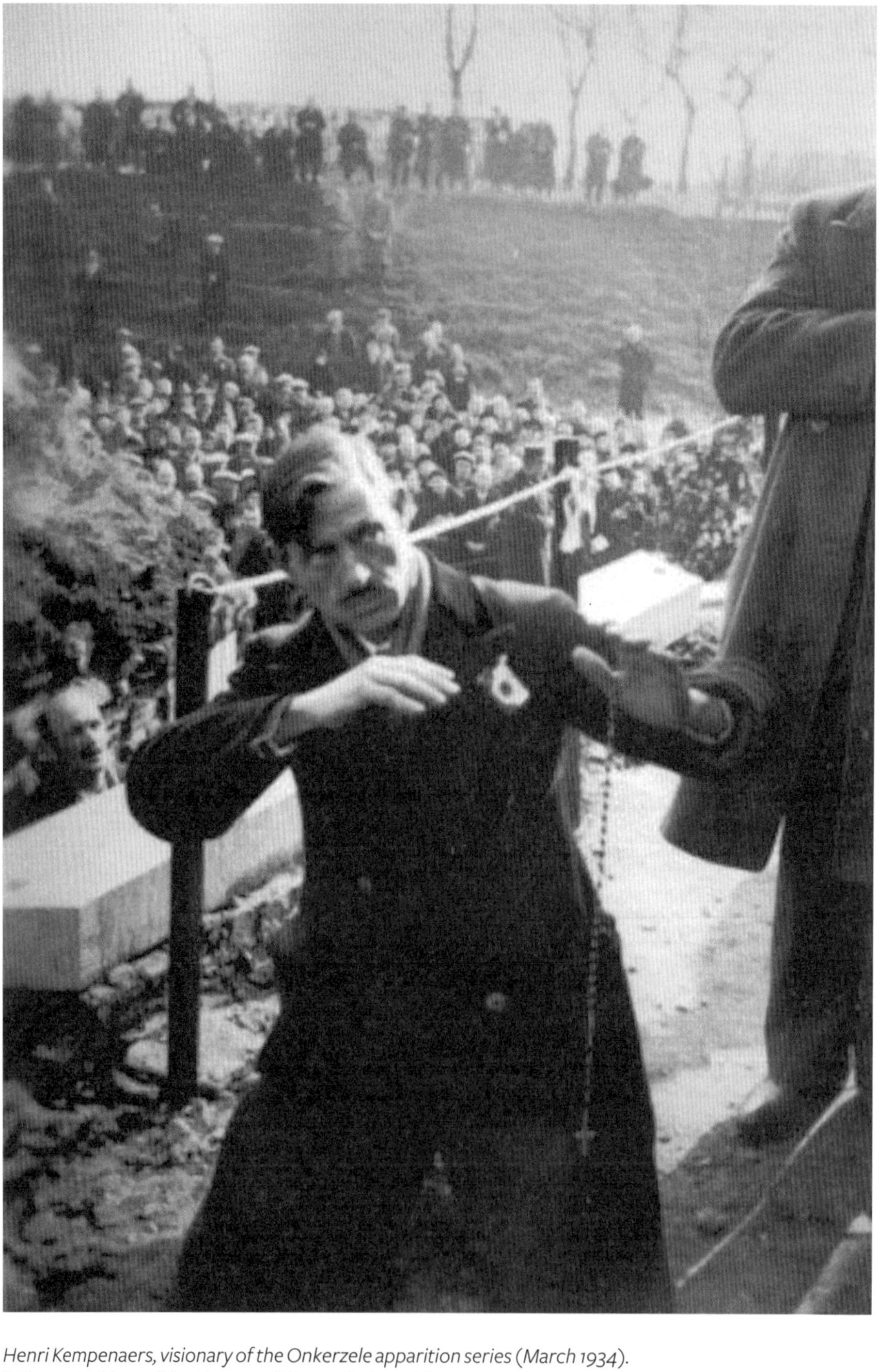

Henri Kempenaers, visionary of the Onkerzele apparition series (March 1934).
[*Ghent, Archives of the Diocese of Ghent, Onkerzele*]

Although the supporters approved of the involvement of the doctors, this does not mean that they readily agreed with the nature of the experiments performed at the site. When, on 21 January 1934 (the events A. Martin also referred to), Dr Fransen and his four colleagues used burning coals during an experiment on a visionary, Leon Sebruyns-Desmet noted in his report how witnesses perceived these experiments to be rather dangerous.[41] The bystanders not only criticized the doctors and the experiments at the time, but also contacted the ecclesiastical authorities to file complaints about the experiments, the doctors' lack of impartiality and even their behaviour.[42] Alfred Magain, for example, contacted the bishop to complain about the comportment of Dr Van Acker and Dr Fransen. Magain had sent in several reports on the series of apparitions, providing factual information on what had happened at the site without adding a personal opinion. This time, however, he was not able to do so. For when he entered the Church of Onkerzele on the same day of 21 January 1934, he noticed that the two doctors were chatting disrespectfully during the service. What is more, when they were singing the *Ave Maria*, he reports, Dr Van Acker joined in, doing so in such a 'fantasist' manner that it could only be meant ironically. It seems that in Magain's opinion their disrespectful behaviour made them less fit for the job they had been asked to carry out. He could think of no excuse for their behaviour.[43]

41 AAM, Processus, B IXa2 (6/1-31/3/1934): Report by Sebruyns-Desmet, 21 January 1934. The experiments performed a year before, on 8 December 1932, during the Beauraing apparitions, seemed to have incited similar responses. When the child visionaries heard about these during the questioning, they refused to be tested again in the same manner. Dr Raymond Leurquin (from Houyet), who testified to the Diocesan Commission on 15 November 1935 about their response, believed that this negative response had a lot to do with the exaggerated way in which the children were told about the tests. ACDF, Dev. Var., Beauraing: 1933.2 (794/1933), box 4: Session 32 (15 November 1935) of the Diocesan Commission of Namur, testimony of Dr Raymond Leurquin.

42 On 19 February, Louis Wilmet contacted the bishop of Ghent and commented on the conduct of Dr Fransen at the Onkerzele site on 1 February 1934. In his opinion, Dr Fransen started his experiments (touching the eye of the visionary with a pencil) even before the visionary went into ecstasy. '... impressionnabilité et de superficialité' ... 'D'où je dois conclure que la commission, loin de faire des conquêtes IMPARTIALES, a d'ores et déjà DÉCIDÉ ET CONCLU, DONC PRÉJUGE ... et elle a le cynisme de le proclamer partout'. AAM, Processus, B IXa1: Wilmet to Coppieters, 19 February 1934. He sent a report on 16 February 1934, and included his letter to Lenain, S.J.

43 AAM, Processus, B IXa2 (6/1-31/3/1934): Report by Alfred Magain on 21 January 1934.

Questioning the manner of questioning

The doctors' experiments triggered reactions, but so did their questioning of the visionaries.[44] In his report about the Onkerzele events of 21 January 1934, Jozef Verbeke also complained about Dr Van Acker. In his opinion, the doctor's behaviour on that day was not professional and far from friendly and it lowered the respect Verbeke and others had for those people who were 'so famous in the intellectual world'. Their dispute that day illuminates Verbeke's limited trust in the competence and expertise of the doctors in religious matters. When the doctor went on endlessly about the visionaries' distraction during the Hail Marys, Verbeke – irritated – responded that no one, even if they had seen the Virgin, would be able to recite two Hail Marys without being the least distracted. Annoyed by the interruption, the doctor asked him about his field of competence. At the time, Verbeke was hindered from answering him, but he wrote in his report what he would have liked to say: 'My competence is that of a convinced Catholic housefather of 15 children, of which two [are] with the good Lord, by all kinds of trials purified, and as far as praying is concerned at least as competent as whatever doctor in medicine, in whose competence this surely does not lie.'[45]

Emphasizing the importance of medical examinations

Although the supporters criticized the way in which the interrogations and tests were done, the doctors' presence at the sites was not under discussion. Apart from enabling doctors to witness the events close up and attend the interrogations,[46] the laypeople also formalized the doctors' involvement (in the examination of the apparitions as well as the miraculous cures), referred to their statements and even imitated their experiments when there was no 'expert' around.

44 AAM, Processus, B IXa2 (6/1-31/3/1934): Report by Alfred Magain on 21 January 1934. It was not only at the Flemish sites that doctors were criticized for their manner of questioning their subjects. The same was said of the doctors who questioned the child visionaries of Beauraing. There were comments about their use of difficult words and phrasings, making it hard for the children to understand what they were being asked and thus making an adequate answer practically impossible, ACDF, Dev. Var., Beauraing: 1933.2 (794/1933), box 4: Session 24 (27 September 1935) of the Diocesan Commission of Namur.

45 AAM, Processus, B IXa2 (6/1-31/3/1934): Testimony of Jozef Verbeke (Etterbeek): '... in de intellectuele wereld zo beroemd' ... 'Mijn competentie is deze van een overtuigd katholieke huisvader van 15 kinderen, waarvan twee bij O.L.Heer, door alle soorten van beproevingen, God zij dank gelouterd, en in zaken bidden zeker zoo bevoegd dan gelijk welke Docter in de medicijnen, in wiens bevoegdheid dit zeker niet ligt.'

46 ACDF, Dev. Var., Beauraing: 1933.2 (794/1933), box 4: Session 65 (3 April 1936) of the Diocesan Commission of Namur. Hector Voisin once stopped a certain Pierre Georges from attending the questioning. He posed as a doctor of science, whereas only doctors in medicine were admitted.

Miraculous cures were considered 'testable', contrary to other types of 'favour', such as temporal favours (job offers, winning the lottery) and the conversions which did not offer similar 'evidence'.[47] The supporters of the site took their cue from Lourdes, where the medical bureau had been established and collected medical reports to support their cases.[48] In the case of Beauraing, this interest resulted in standardized documents to be filled in whenever an exceptional cure took place.[49] The questions on this standard document asked for information about the evolution of the illness: familial antecedents, the doctor in charge, and also referred to a first and a second examination. In addition, the document asked whether there had already been an amelioration before the cure and whether or not the cure could have been caused by the use of medication or have occurred through a natural process. Apart from this questionnaire, the file had to include medical reports that were approved of by the Pro Maria committee (the lay committee in charge of the apparition site).

Interestingly, most of the records that have been preserved in Beauraing are linked to the apparitions of 5 August 1933; that is, the apparitions of Tilman Côme, the adult visionary of Beauraing who was never officially recognized. The same kind of reasoning – the quest for medically approved cases – was at work when the Beauraing Pro Maria committee started to collect doctors' certificates in August-September 1935. To have the first series of Beauraing apparitions approved, they searched for 'credible', that is, medically documented, miracles.[50] A similar interest in medical certificates can be noted at the Flemish sites. Jan Boon, for example, sent the medical reports of sick children – whom the Virgin had promised to heal – to the head of the Medical Society of Saint Luc (they were never cured).[51]

The importance of medical examinations also speaks from the reports on miraculous cures published in the periodicals that were linked to the apparition sites. When we more closely consider the list published in the periodical *Banneux Notre-Dame* on the 1934 cures linked to the Banneux apparitions (early 1933), it is remarkable how much care is taken in reporting on the illness. There are some general descriptions, such as illness ('maladie'), but most of the time the affliction is mentioned in detail: 'Pott's disease' ('mal de pott');

47 ADN, L.42, Wilmet I: Wilmet (?) to Muylle, 10 September 1936.
48 Ibid.: Medical report sent by Dr Gouy, August 1933.
49 ASB, 44, Guérisons et faveurs diverses, on the cure of Hermine Philips-Charlier.
50 ASB, documents of Aurélien Pierroux/Comité Pro Maria, 1934-1935: Letter from the commission asking for the file on the cure of Sr Rose of Mons, 29 August 1935; Ibid.: Letter from the committee to Dr Waszinck of Delft, 17 September 1935, requesting file on the cure of Mme Kersbergen.
51 AAM, Processus, B IIb3: Letter from Jan Boon to Archbishop Van Roey, 20 August 1934. He sent the medical reports of the sick girls of Lokeren to S. Vermeulen, S.J., head of the Medical Society of Saint Luc.

'burning tenosynovitis of the right index finger' ('tenosynovite fougueuse de l'index droit'), 'cephalalgy' ('céphalalgie'), 'pyelitis' ('pyélite'). It seems as if mentioning these details gave extra importance to the cure: an indication that those investigating knew exactly what had been amiss and did not ascribe miraculous qualities to the disappearance of a vague phenomenon that could have healed without the intervention of Mary. Moreover, mentioning the precise term suggested that one had visited a doctor, who had diagnosed the illness or affliction and had not been able to offer a sufficient cure. As Suzanne Kaufman has noted about the miraculous cures in Lourdes, this involvement of modern medicine and the medical narratives that developed 'also made the cures themselves more spectacular'.[52]

More general descriptions were used in the evaluation of the visionaries involved in the Belgian series of apparitions. The lay commentators seem to be well aware that apparitions and related phenomena such as stigmata were linked to hysteria and hallucinations, even though they questioned the credibility of certain descriptions of the visionaries as 'hysterical'[53] and 'hallucinating'[54] on more than one occasion. Most often, these reports refer to the female visionaries, but similar remarks were made about the men.[55] In other words, the bystanders seem to be well aware that visions and cures were not only considered to be the domain of religion and that medical findings could contribute to building stronger cases and/or to condemning others. This generalized 'medical knowledge' influenced the way in which the contemporaries talked about the apparitions and criticized them. What is more, the lay commentators not only adopted the vocabulary, they also seem to be aware of relevant tests.[56]

It is not clear where those laypeople who conducted tests picked up this knowledge: whether they had seen the doctors who were present at the sites perform these tests or whether they knew about them from reports on other apparitions. Whatever the case, in the absence of doctors, some of the bystanders started to do the tests themselves. Most of these tests were done to find out whether or not the visionaries were really in a state of ecstasy. A newspaper article dated 24 September 1933 reports how the people present at the

52 Kaufman, *Consuming Visions*, 96.

53 Archives of the Diocese of Liège (ADL), 30. Banneux, II. Tilman Côme: Letter from M. de Croÿ to abbé, s.d.; PAO, 242. E. C. 4. Laymen: Report by Louis Wilmet, 24 February 1934.

54 ASB, 3, unpublished manuscripts, E: Report of A. Pierroux, 1932-1943.

55 AAM, Processus, B XII.3. Documenta G Varia: Letter of Dewinter, 7 December 1933; PAO, 64, III. B. 9: Report about 23 February 1934, s.n.

56 Sarasin, 'Was ist Wissensgeschichte', 164: '... dass Wissen in seinem "Funktionieren" auf Zirkulation angewiesen ist, dass es auf "Anstöße" aus anderen Wissensfeldern aus unterschiedlichen sozialen Räumen reagiert, an anderen Orten wieder aufgegriffen und dabei umgeformt wird'.

sites had 'voluntarily' carried out some tests themselves that might be of use later on.[57] Similarly, it was reported that the spectators shone flashlights into the eyes of the Onkerzele visionaries, Berthonia and Martha, on 21 November 1933.[58] Both tests seem to have had no effect on the visionaries.

Evaluating the doctors

What happened when it became clear that the doctors' opinion (either positive or negative) did not match the ideas that these laypeople had about the events? How did they minimize the importance of the medical investigations, a significance they themselves had helped to create?

How to interpret medical opinions

The doctors' interest and their involvement at the sites were well known to the general public due to the extensive journalistic coverage of the events. From the first series of apparitions onwards, journalists were present at the sites and published what they believed to be the opinion of the doctors who examined the cases. The evolution of the reports in *De Standaard*, a Catholic Belgian newspaper, is particularly interesting in this respect. Briefly summarized, we can detect the following phases:

(1) In a first phase, the doctors were referred to as personifications of medical authority. On 20 December 1932, *De Standaard* mentioned that Dr Etienne De Greeff and Dr Rouvroy had intensely questioned the child visionaries of Beauraing and considered several explanations: they excluded fraud, but left the possibility open that what had happened might have been a response to nervous shock.[59] The next month, January 1933, the same paper published an article emphasizing how impressed even non-Catholic doctors were:

57 'Te Onkerzele', *De Standaard*, 24 September 1933, 3: 'Vrijwillig zijn door de aanwezigen volksche proefnemingen gedaan welke dan toch van belang kunnen geweest zijn'. For example, on 26 August 1933, a bystander pinched Leonie hard during her apparition. PAO, 86, III. B. 13: Report on the apparitions by Van der Maeren, 4 August -23 September 1933.

58 'Iemand', AAM, Processus c, B IX.A. 1 (19/10-28/12/1933): Report by Magain about Onkerzele on 21 November 1933.

59 'Nog wat over de gebeurtenissen te Beauraing', *De Standaard*, 20 December 1932, 2, provides a short summary of comments by Dr De Greeff and Dr Rouvroy.

> We can add that several witnesses, doctors in medicine, who are not Catholic, have stated that they are strongly impressed by the comportment of the children during ecstasy. They are in agreement in admitting that – without even the slightest hint at believing in a miracle – this comportment in no way belongs to the field of psychiatry as far as that science has developed.[60]

(2) A second phase began when it became clear that the opinion of some of these doctors differed from that of the star reporter for *De Standaard*, Jan Boon. This led Boon to adopt a double strategy: firstly, he did not really question their capacity to make a statement as a doctor, but he did criticize the quality of their research. Secondly, he minimized the importance of the opinions of single doctors and emphasized that in the end it was up to the Church to decide whether or not the apparitions were to be approved. On 12 January 1933, *De Standaard* reported that most of the doctors were astonished by the phenomena and the only natural explanation they could think of related to psychology. Their examinations, however, lacked quality, Jan Boon noted. Regarding Dr August Ladon, he added:

> I am looking for people or facts that may contradict the probability of the supernatural reality of what is happening in Beauraing; time and again, however, I stumble upon mistakes or falsehoods. The study by Dr August Ladon is also riddled with mistakes in the rendition of the facts.

For example, Ladon referred to a miracle that had never been promised and he could not give a scientific explanation for the simultaneity of the children's response to Mary's words or the change in their voices during the apparition.[61] Two months later, the work of Dr De Greeff did not fare any better:

60 'De wonderbare feiten te Beauraing', *De Standaard*, 1-2 January 1933, 2: 'Voegen wij hierbij dat verscheidene getuigen, dokters in de geneeskunde, die niet katholiek geloovig zijn, verklaard hebben sterk onder den indruk te zijn van de houding der kinderen in extase. Ze zijn het trouwens eens om te erkennen – zonder ook maar in 't minst aan een mirakel te gelooven – dat deze houding op geenerlei wijze tot het domein der psychiatrie behoort voor zover deze wetenschap is gevorderd.'

61 J.B., 'De kinderen van Beauraing. Uitputting van natuurlijke opheldering der feiten', *De Standaard*, 12 January 1933, 1: 'Ik zoek personen of feiten die de waarschijnlijkheid van de bovennatuurlijke realiteit van het gebeurde te Beauraing tegenspreken, maar telkens bots ik op vergissingen of onwaarheden. Ook in de studie van Dr. Aug. Ladon wemelt het van fouten bij de weergave der feiten.'

> There is no more conclusive evidence of the frivolity and the annoyingly bad information used by certain medical doctors against Beauraing in the construction of a thesis of their own, than the two exposés that have just appeared in 'Études Carmélitaines (mystiques et missionaires)', written by Prof. Etienne De Greeff and Prof. Van Gehuchten. The latter has hardly spent time in Beauraing ('j'ai très peu vu': I have seen very little), as he himself admitted, since he only paid a short visit to Beauraing. Otherwise, even a low-ranked journalist would not commit the huge errors in reportage that are so numerous in the exposé of Prof. Degreef (sic).[62]

Half a year later, in August 1933, *De Standaard* summarized the opinion of Dr Goedseels, the secretary of the Medical Society of Saint Luc, noting that Goedseels did not believe in the apparitions seen by Tilman Côme (a visionary of Beauraing), and that he had called it theatre and suggested that neuropathy was at work.[63] Jan Boon, again author of the article, added:

> However, the worth of this statement is limited: it is a personal note of doctor Goodsels (sic). 1. The Medical Society of Saint Luc has not yet dedicated a discussion to the case of Tilman Côme; 2. medical doctors do not have any authority, even any competence, to give a verdict about the supernatural character of the apparitions. This authority and competence lie solely with the Church. The bishop of Namur has not yet given a verdict; the ecclesiastical judges have not yet been asked for a decision.[64]

62 J.B., 'De kroniek van Beauraing', *De Standaard*, 19 March 1933, 3: 'Geen doorslaander bewijs van de lichtzinnigheid, en de ergerlijk slechte informatie, welke door zekere geneeskundigen tegenover Beauraing wordt gebruikt voor het opbouwen van een eigen thesis, dan de twee uiteenzettingen zoo pas verschenen in de 'Études Carmélitaines (mystiques et missionaires)' van de hand van Prof. Etienne De Greeff en van Prof. Van Gehuchten. Deze laatste is ternauwernood te Beauraing geweest ('j'ai très peu vu' ik heb weinig gezien) erkende hij zelf daar hij slechts een vluchtig bezoekje bracht te Beauraing. Anderzijds, zelfs een tiende-rangsch journalist zou nog niet de grove reportage onnauwkeurigheden begaan waarvan het opstel van prof. Degreef (sic) krioelt.' See also the introduction to an article a few days later: J.B., 'Beaurang en Banneux. Verschijningen van O.L. Vrouw te Banneux in het bisdom Luik', *De Standaard*, 23 March 1933, 1-2.

63 J.B., 'Naar aanleiding van 5 Augustus te Beauraing. Een gewetensvol enkwest omtrent het geval Tilman Côme', *De Standaard*, 3 August 1933, 1-2, 1.

64 Ibid.: 'De waarde van deze verzekering is echter beperkt: het is een persoonlijke nota van dokter Goodsels. (sic.) 1° de Société Médicale Saint-Luc heeft nog geen enkele beraadslaging gewijd aan de zaak Tilman Côme; 2° geneesheeren hebben geenerlei gezag, zelfs geen bevoegdheid, om uitspraak te doen over het bovennatuurlijk karakter van verschijningen. Dit gezag en deze bevoegdheid behooren uitsluitend aan de Kerk. De bisschop van Namen heeft nog geen oordeel geveld, de kerkelijke rechters is nog niet om een uitspraak gevraagd.'

The articles he published about the medical involvement follow the line of his more private reports, which he sent to the bishops and to other advocates. Similar arguments can also be found among other supporters of apparition sites: they emphasized the lack of scientific character of the doctors' articles in *Les Études*, their circular reasoning and insufficient research.[65] Above all, they criticized the lack of consensus among the doctors. Since every one of them had a different opinion, they could not make claims about the truth of what they were saying – the 'verifiable' reality. Their openness about this only contributed to their vulnerability to criticism.

Nonetheless, in addition to this rather negative 'translation' of the doctors' opinions, there was also a more favourable response to their examinations and hypotheses. C. Derselle's, *La vérité en marche de nouveau*, for example, was a popularized version of the 'blue book' (the articles of *Les Études Carmélitaines*).[66] This was Derselle's second book on the apparition series. His first book on Beauraing, *Et si c'était le Diable?*, had caused a lot of commotion and in this second book he referred to the 'blue book' in order to prove that his criticism had not been so far-fetched.[67]

Derselle started by emphasizing the authority of the authors in question:

> Let us remark first of all that the three above-mentioned authors have, in their specialty, a first-rate competence. As a result, their opinion has a lot more worth than that of all the occasional journalists who thought it necessary to give or even impose their opinion in this affair.[68]

He then contrasted their expertise with that of Dr Maistriaux, the local doctor who was the first to publish on Beauraing:

65 ASB, Comité Pro Maria, 1932-1933: Letter from D. Planque, 13 April 1934 to Mr Nicaise; Ibid., 1934-1935, 171 and 174: Comments on *Les Études*; Ibid., 11. Papers of Gaston Maes, 13: Dossier Planque 'Les années obscures 1935-1943'; ADN, L.2 : Notes Pierroux, 13 March 1936. See also a series of articles in *La Revue Catholique des Idées et les Faits* (by Schyrgens) and the book by Nicaise-Vermer, *Apparitions de la Vierge à Beauraing*.

66 *Études Carmélitaines* also published 'Notre réponse' in 1934 with, among others, a text by Dr De Greeff. *Het Vlaamsch Geneeskundig Tijdschrift*, 10 June 1933, also published on Beauraing.

67 ACDF, Beauraing: 1933.2 (794/1933), box 4: Session 34 (22 November 1935) of the Diocesan Commission of Namur, Dr Derselle will withdraw them, he did not write them, but lent his name; and session 37 (29 November 1935), abbé Derselle wrote them with Dr de Silenrieux, Mr Collard, Melle Van Schingen, Mr le Greffier Van Schingen, abbé Turlot and Dr de Roeck.

68 Derselle, *Beauraing*, 10 : 'Notons d'abord que les trois auteurs prénommés sont, dans leur spécialité, des compétences de tout premier ordre. Par conséquent, leur opinion a une valeur autrement considérable que celle de tous les publicistes d'occasion qui ont prétendu coûté donner et même imposer leur avis en cette affaire.'

> Did Dr Maistriaux have the necessary capacities, or if one wants to put it otherwise, the required professional education, to embark, with a serious chance of succeeding, on the study of a problem as complex as Beauraing? No! He even admitted that himself on 11 December before the doctors De Greeff and Rouvroy.[69]

While none of the doctors involved had first-hand experience with Marian apparitions, some were believed to be better trained to study them. A telling example is the comment made by a visionary from Etikhove. While his behaviour was monitored by local doctors, he complained that he would like to be examined by 'great' doctors: 'I would like to be examined by great doctors. Who knows, maybe I have an illness that makes me act and see this way.' The journalist who noted this comment, added: 'since the visionary himself wishes it, such an examination by psychiatrics and other specialists is certainly not out of place. That man has the right to such an examination, also in the interest of our holy religion.'[70]

Doctors' authority and competence

Competence, authority and capacities were thus central aspects in the discussions for and against – and not solely in the printed press. Aurélien Pierroux, a leading figure in the Pro Maria committee of Beauraing,[71] noted how on 31 December 1932 a discussion developed between the doctors and other bystanders. One of the lay onlookers noted that the 'time for experiments' had passed: 'If the doctors were to have seen something they have had plenty of time, since it has been going on for more than a month, yet their science has not been

69 Derselle, *Beauraing*, 30: 'Le Dr Maistriaux avait-il les capacités nécessaires, ou si l'on veut, la formation professionnelle requisse, pour aborder, avec chance sérieuse d'aboutir, l'étude d'un problème aussi complexe de celui de Beauraing? Non! Il le reconnaît d'ailleurs lui-même, le 11 décembre devant les docteurs De Greeff et Rouvroy.' However, not all laypeople read the popularized version of the doctors' reports: some also read the original publications – and approved. ADN, L.42, Wilmet III: Letter from Wilmet to Princess de Croÿ, 9 November 1934, approving of the criticism expressed in the new issue of *Les Études*.

70 'Onderzoek te Etikhove', *De Standaard*, 21 October 1933, 3: 'Ik zou willen dat ik door groote doktoors onderzocht werd. Wie weet, heb ik soms geen ziekte, die mij zoo doet handelen en zien. Vermits de ziener het zelf wenscht, ware zulk onderzoek door psychiaters en andere specialisten zeker niet misplaatst. Die man heeft recht op zulk onderzoek, ook in 't belang van onzen heiligen godsdienst. We ondervonden trouwens zelf dat hij tamelijk vatbaar is voor suggestie.'

71 He even described the questioning of the visionaries as the task of convinced laypeople rather than as the sole competence of the doctors. ADN, L.2: Notes Pierroux, 13 March 1936.

able to find fault with the little ones.'[72] Likewise, in July 1933, a commentator from Hamont noted that he believed that far too much attention was given to the opinion of the doctors, just as had been the case with Therese Neumann. 'They so readily invoke suggestion, hallucination, hysteria, hypnotism ... the doctors are a little ... materialistic. One consults medical science too much, when it is exactly this which God and the Holy Virgin turn upside-down.'[73] Jozef Verbeke, who, as indicated above, believed himself to be as competent as the doctors in making statements about prayer, even commented that after discussions with several 'intellectuals' he had come to the conclusion that in these series of apparitions:

> ... common sense is worth much more than the thoughts of all these great minds, who attach too much importance to science and, almost always out of pride, pay no attention to spiritual matters, and this is also the case among the Catholics: I have heard more than one Catholic doctor say that there are no miracles happening in Lourdes.[74]

Medical expertise, although welcomed, had its limits, or, as one commentator noted: 'Too much science, decidedly, harms good sense. The man in the street is a better judge in the affair.'[75]

When we take a closer look at the reception of the medical commission – established after all by the ecclesiastical authorities – it becomes clear that the commentators never questioned the reason for its existence (Jan Boon even sent them his reports on Tilman Côme).[76] They did, however, question its ap-

72 ADN, L.2: Notes Pierroux, 13 March 1936: 'Si les médecins avaient dû y voir quelque chose, ils ont eu assez de temps depuis plus d'un mois que cela dure et leur science n'a pu mettre ces petits en défaut. Le temps des expériences est passé.'

73 ASB, documents of A. Pierroux, 1932-1933: Letter from Hamont, 14 July 1933: 'Ils invoquent si facilement la suggestion, hallucination, hystérie, hypnotisme ... Les médecins sont tous un peu ... matérialistes. On consulte trop la science médicale que Dieu ou la Sainte Vierge viennent précisément bouleverser.'

74 AAM, Processus, B IXa2 (6/1-31/3/1934): Jozef Verbeke to Mgr Coppieters, 21 January 1934: '... heb ik ondervonden dat het gezond verstand veel meer waard is dan de gedachten van al die grote geleerden die veel te veel belang hechten aan de wetenschap, en bijna altijd uit hoogmoed geestelijke zaken zonder belang vinden, en dit even veel bij de katholieken, meer dan een katholieke geneesheer heb ik hooren zeggen dat ook te Lourdes geen mirakelen gebeuren.'

75 E.g. Paul Halflants, 'Beauraing et la psychiatrie', on *Les Études* (s.d., cutting), 7: 'Trop de science, décidément, nuit au bon sens. The man in the street est meilleur juge en l'affaire.'

76 KADOC, Archives of Jan Boon, 5.2.5.2: Letter from Jan Boon to Prof. Fransen, 16 June 1934 (included in letter to Cardinal Van Roey).

proach and the impartiality of its members. Jan Boon, Princess de Croÿ[77] and Louis Wilmet all complained about the commission. The latter was particularly critical when addressing the topic in his letters. Referring to their previous statements on the apparitions in a letter to the bishop of Ghent, Wilmet noted 'that the commission, far from being impartial, has on the contrary already decided and concluded, thus prejudges ... and has the cynicism to proclaim this everywhere'. A similar form of decision-making, so he concluded, would have caused a scandal in court.[78]

It should not come as a surprise then that when the verdict of the medical commission reached Wilmet, he was not very impressed.[79] On 4 November 1934,[80] the commission concluded that none of the miraculous cures was to be accepted and dismissed the Flemish visionaries. In the Banneux case, the commission saw a certain psychological disequilibrium, while the child visionaries of Beauraing seemed to be 'normal – although this was not necessarily a confirmation of the supernatural origin of the apparitions.[81] In the report Wilmet sent to Mgr Heylen on 5 December 1934, he commented on the commission's decisions, following the same reasoning he had used earlier and referring to the members' prejudices and the lack of adequate research; in his opinion, an approach 'unworthy of a medical body as important and supposedly scientific-Catholic' as the Medical Society of Saint Luc. In discussing Dr Gouy, who examined the miraculous cure of Tilman Côme, he added that the good doctor had changed his mind after meeting Prof. Van Gehuchten:

77 ADN, L.42, Wilmet III: Letter from Princess de Croÿ to Wilmet, 18 June 1934: this was on Fransen, who allegedly spread the word in Germany that Onkerzele was rejected, although he knew that it had not yet been announced officially. Similarly, Jan Boon complained that Prof. Fransen only observed the apparitions in Onkerzele for a short while – he came only three or four times during the six months that the Onkerzele series of apparitions lasted, AAM, Processus, B IVb: Letter from Jan Boon to Barette (?), 29 August 1934.

78 AAM, Processus, B IXa1: Wilmet to Coppieters, 19 February 1934: '... que la commission, loin de faire des conquêtes IMPARTIALES, a d'ores et déjà DÉCIDÉ ET CONCLU, DONC PRÉJUGE ... et elle a le cynisme de le proclamer partout.' Reflecting on the medical commission that had been established, Louis Wilmet even wrote to Lenain, S.J. in August 1934 claiming that anyone who had any common sense could not attach any value to the statements of the doctors. He argued that the commission only looked for confirmation of what it had already decided to be true, and that one only had to look at their involvement in court cases to realize that there were *tot capita tot sensus*, ADN, L.42, Wilmet III: Letter from Wilmet to Lenain, 5 August 1934.

79 Similar criticism of the decisions of the medical commission, ADN, L.42, Wilmet III: Wilmet, *L'état actuel de Beauraing*, s.d.

80 ADN, L.2: Supernatural facts and apparitions. Diocesan commission for the recognition of the apparitions of Beauraing, opposition to the apparitions of Beauraing from 29 November 1932 to 3 January 1933.

81 ACDF, Dev. Var., Beauraing 1933.2, 24.b: Report by the medical commission of Saint Luc, 4 November 1934.

petrified by the 'learned professor', he had humbly adopted his opinion.[82] The name and fame of members of the commission could thus – in Wilmet's opinion – make other less eminent doctors change their minds. According to Wilmet, freedom of opinion, impartiality and scientific research were all fictions as far as the medical commission was concerned. The doctors' authority in this matter relied on trust: trust in their competence and objectivity. Thus, undermining these aspects was a way to undermine their authority.[83]

Conclusion

The promoters of the apparitions and miraculous cures cleverly cited the doctors and knew that their involvement was a necessary step on the way towards approval. The same holds true for the opponents, who also referred to medical 'authorities' in order to convince people of their 'truth'.[84] Therefore, both sides, neither of whom could claim any scientific or ecclesiastical authority for themselves, helped to uphold the prominent position the Catholic Church had given to medicine in the evaluation of such phenomena. However, when the doctors publicly formulated their opinions and they did not concur with those of the laymen and women other tactics were put to use. The quality of their examination was brought into question and so was their authority on the matter. In the end, as certain lay commentators emphasized, it was up to the ecclesiastical authorities (and not to doctors) to decide whether or not the series of apparitions were to be accepted and thus whether or not the exceptional corporeal phenomena had a pathological or supernatural origin: whether an exceptional event was truly 'miraculous'.[85]

The more often medical knowledge was called upon, the more it was questioned – a conundrum that Wiebe Bijker, Roland Bal and Ruud Hendriks have called the 'paradox of scientific authority'.[86] In the case of the Belgian series of apparitions, the medical authorities could be questioned by referring

82 ADN, L.42, Wilmet IV: Dossier Côme, sent to Mgr Heylen post 5 December 1934: 'sans examen sérieux de ce cas, avec un parti-pris indigne d'un corps médical aussi important et soi-disant scientifique-catholique'; 'il a été médusé par le "savant professeur" et il s'est humblement rangé à son avis'.

83 Krieger, 'The Idea of Authority', footnote 7.

84 De Certeau, *The Practice of Everyday Life*, 188: 'Citation thus appears to be the ultimate weapon for making people believe. Because it plays on what the other is assumed to believe, it is the means by which the "real" is instituted. To cite the other on their behalf (189) is hence to make credible the simulacra produced in a particular place.'

85 ADN, L5bis: A. Wirix, Apparitions et miracles. Attitude qui convient aux catholiques, 26 February 1933.

86 Bijker, Bal and Hendriks, *The Paradox of Scientific Authority*.

to those who had the final say in the evaluation of the phenomena. In other words, instead of challenging the authority of the Church – a feature often referred to in research on the lay reception of mystical phenomena[87] – laypeople used the hierarchical order to counter the findings of the doctors. Interestingly, the doctors they particularly focused on, the members of the medical commission, had in fact been given a certain authority by the Church.

87 For example, by emphasizing the importance of the personal religious experience. The lack of social power of the visionaries (often from a poor rural background) enhances their credibility. Christian, 'Six Hundred Years of Visionaries in Spain', 118.

BIBLIOGRAPHY

Abbreviations

AAM:	Archives of the Archdiocese of Mechelen-Brussels
ACDF:	Archives of the Congregation for the Doctrine of the Faith
ADL:	Archives of the Diocese of Liège
ADN:	Archives of the Diocese of Namur
ASB:	Archives of the Sanctuary of Beauraing
DCF:	Documentação Crítica de Fátima
HA LKH:	Historisches Archiv des Landeskrankenhauses Hall in Tirol
PAO:	Parish Archives Onkerzele
SHAT:	Service Historique de l'Armée de Terre

Archives

Beauraing, Archives of the Sanctuary of Beauraing (ASB).
Edinburgh, Scottish Catholic Archives.
Fátima, Documentação Crítica de Fátima (DCF).
Ghent, Archives of the Diocese of Ghent.
Hall (Tirol), Historisches Archiv des Landeskrankenhauses Hall in Tirol (HA LKH).
Leuven, KADOC-KU Leuven, Archives Jan Boon.
Liège, Archives of the Diocese of Liège (ADL).
Mechelen, Archives of the Archdiocese of Mechelen-Brussels (AAM).
Namur, Archives of the Diocese of Namur (ADN).
Onkerzele, Parish Archives Onkerzele (PAO).
Vatican City, Archives of the Congregation for the Doctrine of the Faith (ACDF).
Vincennes, Service historique de la Défense: Service Historique de l'Armée de Terre (SHAT).

Published sources and literature

Albert, Jean-Pierre. *Le sang et le ciel. Les saintes mystiques dans le monde chrétien*. S.l.: Aubier, 1997.

Al-Kattani, Muhammad ibn Ja'far. *Kitab Salwat al-anfas wa muhadathat al-akyas bi man uqbira min al-'ulama' wa al-sulaha' bi Fas*. Fez, 1898, 3 vols.

Amiotte-Suchet, Laurent. 'Tous égaux devant Dieu? Réflexions sur les logiques d'éligibilité des miraculés'. *Social Compass*, 52 (2005) 2, 241-254.

Amster, Ellen. *Medicine and the Saints: Science, Islam, and the Colonial Encounter in Morocco, 1877-1956*. Austin: University of Texas Press, 2013.

Annales de Notre-Dame de Lourdes. Published by the RR PP Missionaries of the Immaculate Conception. Lourdes: Bertrand Pujo, 1868-1944.

Apolito, Paolo. *The Internet and the Madonna: Religious Visionary Experience on the Web*. Chicago: University of Chicago Press, 2005.

Araújo, Henrique Gomes de. *Histeria, pithiatismo. Dados teóricos e observações clínicas. Estado actual da questão*. Porto: Livraria Moreira, 1919.

Ashburnham, M. Catherine. 'Letter to the Editor'. *The Tablet*, 29 January 1938, 151.

Bader, Meinrad. *Der alte Fließer Pfarrer. Blätter der Erinnerung an den heiligmäßigen Exorcisten Simon Alois Maaß (1805-1846)*. Innsbruck: Verlag der Kinderfreund-Anstalt, 1899.

Barrère, Joseph. *Berguille, ou l'extatique de Fontet: Apparitions accompagnées de divers prodiges*. Paris: Enault et Vic, 1875.

Bazzaz, Sahar. *Forgotten Saints: History, Power, and Politics in the Making of Modern Morocco*. Cambridge, Mass.: Center for Middle East Studies, Harvard University, 2010.

Bender, Courtney et al. 'Religion on the Move: Mapping Global Cultural Production and Consumption' in: Courtney Bender et al., eds. *Religion on the Edge: De-Centering and Re-Centering the Sociology of Religion*. New York: Oxford University Press, 2013, 159-176.

Benzenhöfer, Udo. *Psychiatrie und Anthropologie in der ersten Hälfte des 19. Jahrhunderts*. Hürtgenwald: Guido Pressler, 1993.

Bijker, Wiebe; Bal, Roland and Hendriks, Ruud. *The Paradox of Scientific Authority: The Role of Scientific Advice in Democracies*. Cambridge: MIT Press, 2009.

Blackbourn, David. *Marpingen: Apparitions of the Virgin Mary in Nineteenth-Century Germany*. New York: Alfred A. Knopf, 1994.

Blasius, Dirk. *Umgang mit Unheilbarem. Studien zur Sozialgeschichte der Psychiatrie*. Bonn: Psychiatrie Verlag, 1986.

Blasius, Dirk. *'Einfache Seelenstörung'. Geschichte der deutschen Psychiatrie 1800-1945*. Frankfurt am Main: Fischer Taschenbuch, 1994.

Boissarie, Gustave. *Lourdes, histoire médicale, 1858-1891*. Paris: V. Lecoffre, 1891.

Boissarie, Gustave. *Lourdes depuis 1858 jusqu'à nos jours*. Paris: Sanard et Derangeon, 1894.

Boissarie, Gustave. *Les grandes guérisons de Lourdes*. Paris: P. Téqui, 1900.

Bonduelle, Michel; Gelfand, Toby and Goetz, Christopher G. *Charcot, un grand médecin dans son siècle*. Paris, 1996 (original in English, 1995).

Borutta, Manuel. 'Das Andere der Moderne. Geschlecht, Sexualität und Krankheit in antikatholischen Diskursen Deutschlands und Italien (1850-1900)' in: Werner Rammert et al. *Kollektive Identitäten und kulturelle Innovationen. Ethnologische, soziologische und historische Studien*. Leipzig: Leipziger Universitätsverlag, 2001, 59-76.

Borutta, Manuel. 'Genealogie der Säkularisierungstheorie. Zur Historisierung einer großen Erzählung der Moderne'. *Geschichte und Gesellschaft*, 36 (2010), 347-376.

Bossant, Els. *Het dossier van de verschijningen te Beauraing: een psychologische analyse en evaluatie*. Diss. Lic. KU Leuven, 1992.

Bouflet, Joachim. 'Avant-propos' in: Antoine Imbert-Gourbeyre. *La stigmatisation*. Grenoble: Éditions Jérôme Million, 1996 (1894), 7-18.

Bouflet, Joachim and Philippe Boutry. *Un signe dans le ciel. Les apparitions de la Vierge*. Paris: Bernard Grasset, 1997.

Bourdin, Dr. *L'extatique de Fontet. Extrait des Annales médico-psychologiques*. Paris: Imprimerie de E. Donnaud, 1878.

Bowman, F.P. 'Une lecture politique de la folie religieuse ou 'théomanie''. *Romantisme*, 24 (1979), 75-87.

Brockmeyer, Bettina. *Selbstverständnisse. Dialoge über Körper und Gemüt im frühen 19. Jahrhundert*. Göttingen: Wallstein Verlag, 2009.

Brumberg, Joan Jacobs. *Fasting Girls: The Emergence of Anorexia as a Modern Disease*. Cambridge: Harvard University Press, 1988.

Burton, Richard D.E. *Holy Tears, Holy Blood: Women, Catholicism, and the Culture of Suffering in France, 1840-1970*. Ithaca: Cornell University Press, 2004.

Bynum, Caroline. 'Holy Anorexia in Modern Portugal'. *Culture, Medicine and Psychiatry*, 12 (1988), 239-248.

Cabral, João de Pina. *Sons of Adam, Daughters of Eve*. Oxford: Clarendon Press, 1986.

Cahill, M. 'Teresa Higginson'. *The Tablet*, 18 December 1937, 848.

Cammack, James S. 'Letter to the Editor'. *The Tablet*, 22 January 1938, 118.

Cammack, James S. 'Letter to the Editor'. *The Tablet*, 5 February 1938, 174.

Cammack, James S. *Moral Problems of Mental Defect*. London: Burns & Oates, 1938.

Campana, E. 'Gratitude to Teresa Higginson'. *The Tablet*, 4 December 1937, 754.

Campana, E. 'Letter to the Editor'. *The Tablet*, 22 January 1938, 121.

Capes, Harriet M. and McNabb, Vincent, eds. *The Life of Father Bertrand Wilberforce, O.P.* London / Edinburgh: Sands & Co., 1906.

Carroy, Jacqueline. *Le mal de Morzine: De la possession à l'hystérie (1857-1877)*. Paris: Solin, 1981.

Cartmell, J. 'Notes on Recent Work. Ascetical and Mystical Theology'. *The Clergy Review*, 13 (1937) 2, 93-97.

Carvalho, David Luna de. *Os Levantes da República (1910-1917): Resistências à laicização e movimentos populares de repertório tradicional na 1ª República*. Porto: Edições Afrontamento, 2011.

Le cas de De Rudder devant les médecins. Bibliothèque de Propagande, XI.1. Brussels, 1913.

Casselman, Joris. *Etienne De Greeff, 1898-1961. Psychiater, criminoloog en romanschrijver. Leven, werk en huidige betekenis*. Antwerp: Maklu, 2010.

'The Catholic Medical Guild'. *The Tablet*, 26 October 1935, 18.

'A Catholic Psychological Society'. *The Tablet*, 30 November 1935, 23.

'Catholic Psychological Society. A Lecture on Freud'. *The Tablet*, 3 April 1937, 490-491.

Chabauty, Emmanuel-A. *Les prophéties modernes vengées ou la défense de la concordance de toutes les prophéties*. Poitiers: H. Oudin and Paris: V. Palmé, 1874.

Charcot, Jean-Martin. 'La foi qui guérit'. *Revue hebdomadaire*, (1892) 5, 112-132. First published in English: 'Faith Cure'. *New Review*, (1892) 11, 244-262.

Charcot, Jean-Martin and Richer, Paul. *Les démoniaques dans l'art*. Paris: A. Delahaye and E. Lecrosnier, 1887.

Charcot, Jean-Martin and Richer, Paul. *Les démoniaques dans l'art*, followed by Jean-Martin Charcot. *La foi qui guérit*. Paris: Macula, 1984.

Charlier, Jean-Michel. *Léon Degrelle: persiste et signe. Interviews recueillies pour la télévision française par Jean-Michel Charlier*. Paris: Picollec, 1985.

Chiron, Yves. *Enquête sur les apparitions de la Vierge*. Paris: Perrin and Mame, 1995 (first edition); Paris: Perrin, 1997; 2007.

Chmielewski, Alexandra. 'Norm und Autonomie. Legitimierungsstrategien und Deutungsmacht süddeutscher Anstaltspsychiater in der ersten Hälfte des 19. Jahrhunderts" in: Heiner Fangerau and Karen Nolte, eds. *"Moderne" Anstaltspsychiatrie im 19. und 20. Jahrhundert – Legitimation und Kritik*. Stuttgart: Franz Steiner Verlag, 2006, 67-82.

Christian, William. 'L'œil de l'esprit. Les visionnaires basques en transe, 1931'. *Terrain*, 30 (1998), 5-22.

Christian, William. 'Six Hundred Years of Visionaries in Spain: Those Believed and Those Ignored' in: Michael Hanagan, Leslie Page Moch and Wayne te Brake, eds. *Challenging Authority: The Historical Study of Contentious Politics*. Minneapolis/London: University of Minnesota Press, 1998, 107-119.

Claeys Boúúaert, M. 'C. Kerr, *Theresia Helena Higginson ou la vie merveilleuse d'une institutrice libre anglaise*, tr. par V. Billé'. *Nouvelle revue théologique*, 63 (November 1936) 9, 1088.

Clauchai-Larsenal, Charles. *Berguille et Louise Lateau. Étude comparative*. Bordeaux: L. Coderc, 1874.

Clauchai-Larsenal, Charles. *Pourquoi je crois à Berguille! Réponse au Rosier de Marie et à M.V. de Portets*. Bordeaux: L. Coderc, 1874.

Clifford, James. *The Predicament of Culture: Twentieth-Century Ethnography, Literature and Art*. Cambridge, Mass.: Harvard University Press, 1988.

Clifford, James and Marcus, George, eds. *Writing Culture: The Poetics and Politics of Ethnography*. Berkeley: University of California Press, 1986.

Cohen, Lizabeth. 'Re-Viewing the Twentieth Century through an American Catholic Lens' in: R. Scott Appleby and Kathleen Sprows Cummings, eds. *Catholics in the American Century: Recasting Narratives of U.S. History*. Ithaca: Cornell University Press, 2012, 43-60.

Cornell, Vincent. *Realm of the Saint: Power and Authority in Moroccan Sufism*. Austin: University of Texas Press, 1998.

Corrado Pope, Barbara. 'Immaculate and Powerful: The Marian Revival in the Nineteenth Century' in: Clarissa W. Atkinson, Constance H. Buchanan and Margaret R. Miles, eds. *Immaculate and Powerful: Female in Sacred Image and Social Reality*. Boston: Beacon Press, 1985, 173-200.

Costa, Alexandrina. *Autobiografia*. <http://alexandrinabalasar.free.fr/autobiografia_2.htm>.

Cox, Jeffrey. 'Secularization and Other Master Narratives of Religion in Modern Europe'. *Kirchliche Zeitgeschichte*, 14 (2001), 24-35.

Crapanzano, Vincent. *The Hamadsha: A Study in Moroccan Ethnopsychiatry*. Berkeley / Los Angeles: University of California Press, 1973.

Csordas, Thomas. *Body/Meaning/Healing*. New York: Palgrave Mcmillan, 2002.

Cummings, Kathleen Sprows. 'American Saints: Gender and the Re-Imaging of U.S. Catholicism in the Early Twentieth Century'. *Religion & American Culture: A Journal of Interpretation*, 22 (2012) 2, 203-231.

Curicque, Jean-Marie. *Voix prophétiques ou signes, apparitions et prédictions modernes*. Paris: Victor Palmé, 1872, 2 vols.

Curran, Emmet. '"The Finger of God is Here": The Advent of the Miraculous in the Nineteenth-Century American Catholic Community'. *Catholic Historical Review*, 73 (1987) 1, 41-61.

Daston, Lorraine and Galison, Peter. *Objectivity*. New York: Zone Books, 2007.

Daston, Lorraine and Lunbeck, Elizabeth. 'Introduction: Observation Observed' in: Lorraine Daston and Elizabeth Lunbeck, eds. *Histories of Scientific Observation*. Chicago: University of Chicago Press, 2011, 1-9.

Daurelle, l'Abbé. *Les évènements de Fontet d'après les principes de St Thomas*. Rome: Imprimerie de Rome, 1878.

Davies, John. 'Traditional Religion, Popular Piety, or Base Superstition? The Cause for the Beatification of Teresa Higginson'. *Recusant History*, 23 (1996-1997), 123-144.

Debreyne, Pierre Jean Corneille. *Essai sur la théologie morale considérée dans ses rapports avec la physiologie et la médecine*. Paris: Poussielgue-Rusang, 1842.

De Certeau, Michel. 'Ce que Freud fait de l'histoire. A propos de 'Une névrose démoniaque au XVIIe siècle''. *Annales, Economies, Sociétés, Civilisations*, 25 (1970) 3, 654-667.

De Certeau, Michel. *The Practice of Everyday Life*. Berkeley: University of California Press, 1988 (first edition 1984).

De Giorgio, Michela. 'Die Gläubige' in: Ute Frevert and Heinz-Gerhard Haupt, eds. *Der Mensch des 19. Jahrhunderts*. Frankfurt am Main / New York: Campus, 1999, 120-147.

De Meester, Alphonsus. *La guérison miraculeuse de Pierre De Rudder. Relation des deux premières enquêtes faites en 1875*. Roulers: De Meester, 1910.

De Meester, Alphonsus. *De wonderbare genezing van Pieter De Rudder. Het kanoniek onderzoek, 1907-1908*. Oostakker: Basiliek van O.-L.-Vrouw van Lourdes, 1957.

Derselle, Clément. *Beauraing. La vérité en marche du nouveau!* Charleroi: Souris F. & Ribaux, 1933.

Deschamps, Alfred. *Le cas de Pierre De Rudder et les objections des médecins. Monographie d'un miracle de Lourdes-Oostakker*. Brussels: Librairie de l'Action catholique, 1913.

Desmazières, Agnes. 'Psychology against Medicine? Mysticism in the Light of Scientific Apologetics'. *Revue belge de philologie et d'histoire*, 88 (2010), 1191-1212.

Desmazières, Agnès. *L'Inconscient au paradis. Comment les catholiques ont reçu la psychanalyse (1920-1965)*. Paris: Payot & Rivages, 2011.

Deville, M. *Notice historique sur la dévotion de Notre-Dame des Anges établie dans la paroisse de Pouvourville*. Toulouse: Imprimerie de Bonnal & Gibrac, 1871.

Devlin, Judith. *The Superstitious Mind: French Peasants and the Supernatural in the Nineteenth Century*. New Haven: Yale University Press, 1987.

Didi-Huberman, Georges. *Invention de l'hystérie. Charcot et l'iconographie photographique de la Salpêtrière*. Paris: Macula, 1982.

Dols, Michael W. *Majnun: The Madman in Medieval Society*. Oxford: Clarendon Press, 1992.

Doutté, Edmond. 'Notes sur l'islam maghribin: les marabouts'. *Revue de l'histoire des religions*, 40 (1899), 343-369 and 41 (1899), 289-366.

Doutté, Edmond. *L'Islam algérien en l'an 1900*. Algiers: Giralt, 1900.

Doutté, Edmond. *Les Tas de pierres sacrés et quelques pratiques connexes dans le Sud du Maroc*. Algiers: Imprimerie Administrative Victor Heitz, 1903.

Doutté, Edmond. *Merrâkech*. Paris: Comité du Maroc, 1905.

Doutté, Edmond. *Magie et religion dans l'Afrique du Nord*. Algiers: Jourdan, 1908.

Drouin, Jean-Claude. 'Un légitimiste mystique du XIXème siècle: Adrien Péladan, 1815-1890' in: Jean-Pierre Laurant and Victor Nguyen, eds. *Les Péladan*. Lausanne: Cahiers de l'Herne, 1990, 13-19.

Duffin, Jacalyn. *Medical Miracles: Doctors, Saints, and Healing in the Modern World*. Oxford: Oxford University Press, 2009.

Edelman, Nicole. *Voyantes, guérisseuses et visionnaires: Somnambules et médiums en France, 1795-1914*. Paris: Michal, 1995.

Edelman, Nicole. *Les métamorphoses de l'hystérique. Du début du XIXe siècle à la Grande Guerre*. Paris: Éditions La Découverte, 2003.

Elaut, L. 'Mirakel en wetenschap. De beenderen van Pieter De Rudder'. *Universitas Schriften*, (1951) 2, 93-103.

Fairfield, Letitia. 'Letter to the Editor'. *The Tablet*, 12 February 1938, 213-214.

Falleyn, Joanna. *Hysterie en de medische wereld in België, 1855-1914*. Diss. KU Leuven, 1999.

Feierman, Steven. 'Healing as Social Criticism in the Time of Colonial Conquest'. *African Studies*, 54 (1995) 1, 73-88.

Ferrand, Camille. *La vérité touchant Berguille, la voyante de Fontet et les manifestations surnaturelles*. Bordeaux: L. Coderc, 1874.

Ferry, Edmond. *La Réorganisation marocaine (Rapport au Comité du Maroc)*. Paris: Comité du Maroc, 1905.

Finotti, Joseph M., SJ. *The Mystery of the Wizard Clip*. Baltimore, 1879.

Foucault, Michel. *The Birth of the Clinic: An Archaeology of Medical Perception*. New York: Pantheon Books, 1973.

Freud, Sigmund. *Une névrose démoniaque au XVIIe siècle*. Quebec, Chicoutimi: Gallimard, 1933 (translated from German by Marie Bonaparte and Mme E. Marty, 1927. Digital version produced by Jean-Marie Tremblay (Cégep, Chicoutimi): <http://www.uqac.uquebec.ca/zone30/Classiques_des_sciences_sociales/index.html>.

Freud, Sigmund. 'A Seventeenth-Century Demonological Neurosis' in: [James Strachey, ed.] *The Standard Edition of the Complete Psychological Works of Sigmund Freud*. Vol. 19. London: Hogarth Press, 1961, 72-105.

Freud, Sigmund and Josef Breuer. *Studies on Hysteria*. Ed. and tr. James and Alix Strachey. Harmondsworth: Penguin Books, 1974.

Gilley, Sheridan. 'Vulgar Piety and the Brompton Oratory, 1850-1860'. *Durham University Journal*, 43 (1981), 15-21.

Gilman, Sander. *Seeing the Insane: A Visual and Cultural History of Our Attitude towards the Mentally Ill*. New York: John Wiley & Sons, 1982.

Gilman, Sander. 'The Image of the Hysteric' in: Sander Gilman et al., eds. *Hysteria Beyond Freud*. Berkeley: University of California, 1993, 345-452.

Gjerde, Jon. *Catholicism and the Shaping of Nineteenth-Century America*. Ed. S. Deborah Kang. Cambridge: Cambridge University Press, 2012.

Glatzel, Johann. *Melancholie und Wahnsinn. Beiträge zur Psychopathologie und ihre Grenzgebiete*. Darmstadt: Wiss. Buchgesellschaft, 1990.

Goldberg, Ann. *Sex, Religion and the Making of Modern Madness: The Eberbach Asylum and German Society, 1815-1849*. New York: Oxford University Press, 1999.

Goldstein, Jan. 'The Hysteria Diagnosis and the Politics of Anticlericalism in Late Nineteenth-Century France'. *The Journal of Modern History*, 54 (1982) 2, 209-239.

Goldstein, Jan. 'Psychiatry' in: William F. Bynum and Roy Porter. *Companion Encyclopaedia of the History of Medicine*. London: Routledge, 1993, 1350-1372.

Goldstein, Jan. *Console and Classify: The French Psychiatric Profession in the Nineteenth Century*. Cambridge: Cambridge University Press, 1987; Chicago: University of Chicago Press, 2001.

Gordon, Rae Beth. *De Charcot à Charlot. Mises en scène du corps pathologique*. Rennes: Presses Universitaires de Rennes, 2013 (original in English, 2001).

Gowland, Angus. 'The Problem of Early Modern Melancholy'. *Past and Present*, 191 (2006), 77-120.

Une grande inconnue ou, Les merveilles d'une simple vie: Teresa Higginson (1844-1905). Cagnotte, 1953.

Guide national et catholique du voyageur en France. Deuxième partie: Tome II: Réseaux d'Orléans-État et du Midi et lignes de correspondance. Paris: Maison de la bonne presse, 1901.

Guillemain, Hervé. *Diriger les consciences, guérir les âmes. Une histoire comparée des pratiques thérapeutiques et religieuses (1830-1939)*. Paris: La Découverte, 2006.

Guise-Castelnuovo, Antoinette. *Le docteur Boissarie et les 'guéris' de Lourdes face aux experts de la Salpêtrière et de l'école de Nancy (1890-1914)*. Colloquium 'La science par en bas', held at the University of Maine by CERHIO (University of Rennes 2). <http://www.canal-u.tv/?redirectVideo=14414> (7 June 2013).

Harris, Ruth. 'Possession on the Borders: The "Mal de Morzine" in Nineteenth-Century France'. *Journal of Modern History*, 69 (1997), 451-478.

Harris, Ruth. *Lourdes. Body and Spirit in the Secular Age*. New York: Penguin Books, 1999.

Harris, Ruth. *Lourdes. La grande histoire des apparitions, des pèlerinages et des guérisons*. Paris: Éditions Jean-Claude Lattès, 2001.

Harris, Ruth. 'The "unconscious" and Catholicism in France'. *The Historical Journal*, 47 (2004) 2, 331-354.

Harris, Ruth. 'Les miraculées de Lourdes' in: Jacqueline Carroy et al., eds. *Les femmes dans les sciences de l'homme (XIXe-XXe siècles)*. Paris: Seli Arslan, 2005, 287-300.

Hartney, Christopher. 'Finding a Place for Possession, Divination, and Trance within the Historical Perspective'. *Journal of Religious History*, 38 (2014) 2, 263-273.

Hayward, Rhodri. 'Demonology, Neurology and Medicine in Edwardian Britain'. *Bulletin of the History of Medicine*, 78 (2004), 37-58.

Heidegger, Maria. 'Seelsorge in der frühen Anstaltspsychiatrie: Das Beispiel Hall in Tirol im Vormärz'. *Virus. Beiträge zur Sozialgeschichte der Medizin*, 8 (2009), 71-83.

Heidegger, Maria. 'Körper – Seele – Leid. Entäußerungen des Irrsinns in der ärztlichen Wahrnehmung der 1830er Jahre' in: Kordula Schnegg and Elisabeth Grabner-Niel, eds. *Körper er-fassen. Körpererfahrungen, Körpervorstellungen, Körperkonzepte*. Innsbruck/Vienna/Bozen: Studienverlag, 2010, 134-147.

Heidegger, Maria. 'Handlungsräume und Positionen von Anstaltsgeistlichen in der k. k. Provinzial-Irrenanstalt Hall in Tirol (1830-1870)' in: Falk Bretschneider, Martin Scheutz and Alfred Stefan Weiß, eds. *Personal und Insassen von 'totalen Institutionen' - zwischen Konfrontation und Verflechtung*. Leipzig: Universitätsverlag Leipzig, 2011, 271-288.

Heidegger, Maria. 'Die Seelsorger und ihre homöopathische Hausapotheke. Katholische Geistliche als Laienheiler in Tirol im 19. Jahrhundert'. *Virus. Beiträge zur Sozialgeschichte der Medizin*, 13 (2015), 75-92.

Heidegger, Maria and Seifert, Oliver. 'Nun ist aber der Zweck einer Irrenanstalt Heilung. Zur Positionierung des "Irrenhauses" innerhalb der psychiatrischen Landschaft Tirols im 19. und frühen 20. Jahrhundert'. *Geschichte und Region / storia e regione*, 17 (2008) 2, 24-46.

Heimann, Mary. *Catholic Devotion in Victorian England*. Oxford: Oxford University Press, 1995.

Heimann, Mary. 'Herbert Henry Charles Thurston'. *Oxford Dictionary of National Biography*, vol. 54. Oxford: Oxford University Press, 2004, 728-729.

Heimann, Mary. 'Mary Ann Girling'. *Oxford Dictionary of National Biography*, vol. 22. Oxford: Oxford University Press, 2004, 347-348.

Heimann, Mary. 'Teresa Helena Higginson' in: *Oxford Dictionary of National Biography*, vol. 27. Oxford: Oxford University Press, 2004, 71-72.

Heimann, Mary. 'Mysticism in Bootle: Victorian Supernaturalism as an Historical Problem'. *Journal of Ecclesiastical History*, 64 (April 2013), 335-356.

Heinroth, Johann Christian August. *Lehrbuch der Störungen des Seelenlebens oder der Seelenstörungen und ihrer Behandlung. Vom rationalen Standpunkt aus entworfen. Theile 1-2. Mit Anhang: Anweisung für angehende Irrenärzte zu richtiger Behandlung ihrer Kranken*. Leipzig: Fr. Chr. Wilh. Vogel, 1818.

Heinroth, Johann Christian August. *Textbook of Disturbances of Mental Life; or, Disturbances of the Soul and Their Treatments*. Trans. J. Schmorak. Vol. 1: *Theory*. Baltimore: John Hopkins University Press, 1975.

Homerin, Thomas Emil. 'Ibn Taimiya's *Al-Sufiya wa-al-Fuqara*'. *Arabica*, 32 (1985), 219-244.

Honnor, Brian. *Appreciations of Teresa Helena Higginson, School-Teacher and Mystic*. Taunton: n.p., 1986.

Hunt, Linda M. 'Strategic Suffering: Illness Narratives as Social Empowerment among Mexican Cancer Patients' in: Cheryl Mattingly and Linda C. Garro, eds. *Narrative and the Cultural Construction of Illness and Healing*. Berkeley: University of California Press, 2000, 88-107.

Hutchings, Michael, ed. *Teresa Helena Higginson: The Servant of God... The Collection of Papers Concerning the Life and Mission of Teresa Helena Higginson*. London: M.C. Hutchings, 2000.

Hutchinson, William. *Religious Pluralism in America: The Contentious History of a Founding Ideal*. New Haven: Yale University Press, 2003.

Imbert-Gourbeyre, Antoine. *Les Stigmatisées*. Paris: Palmé, 1873, 2 vols.

International Marian Research Institute. <www.udayton.edu/imri>. 'The Mary Page'.

Jackson, Stanley. *Care of the Psyche: A History of Psychological Healing*. New Haven: Yale University Press, 1999.

Jacobi, Walter. *Die Stigmatisierten: Beiträge zur Psychologie der Mystik*. Munich: Verlag von J.F. Bergmann, 1923.

Jansen, Willy and Notermans, Catrien. 'From vision to cult site: A comparative perspective'. *Archives de sciences sociales des religions*, 151 (2010), 71-90.

Janzen, John. *The Quest for Therapy in Lower Zaire*. Berkeley / Los Angeles: University of California Press, 1978.

Johnston, Francis. *Alexandrina: The Agony and The Glory*. Rockford (Illinois): TAN Books and Publishers, 1982.

Jonas, Raymond. *France and the Cult of the Sacred Heart: An Epic Tale for Modern Times*. Berkeley / Los Angeles: University of California Press, 2000.

Joset, Camille-Jean. *Dossiers de Beauraing*. 4: *Sources et documents primitifs inédits antérieurs à la mi-mars 1933*. Namur/Beauraing: Facultés universitaires Notre-Dame de la Paix, 1982.

Joset, Camille-Jean and Toussaint, F. *Beauraing. Les apparitions*. Bar-le-Duc: Desclée-De Brouwer, 1981.

Kane, Paula. '"She offered herself up": The Victim Soul and Victim Spirituality in Catholicism'. *Church History*, 71 (2002) 1, 80-119.

Kane, Paula. *Sister Thorn and Catholic Mysticism in Modern America*. Chapel Hill: University of North Carolina Press, 2013.

Karamustafa, Ahmed. *God's Unruly Friends: Dervish Groups in the Islamic Middle Period, 1200-1550*. Oxford: Oneworld Publications, 2006.

Kaufman, Suzanne. *Consuming Visions: Mass Culture and the Lourdes Shrine*. Ithaca-London: Cornell University Press, 2005.

Kaufmann, Doris. *Aufklärung, bürgerliche Selbsterfahrung und die "Erfindung" der Psychiatrie in Deutschland, 1770-1850*. Göttingen: Vandenhoeck & Ruprecht, 1995.

Keller, Richard. *Colonial Madness: Psychiatry in French North Africa*. Chicago: University of Chicago Press, 2007.

Kelly, Thomas S. 'Letter to the Editor'. *The Tablet*, 25 December 1937, 886.

Kelly, Thomas S. 'Letter to the Editor'. *The Tablet*, 19 February 1938, 247-249.

Kennedy, Grace. *Father Clement: A Roman Catholic Story*. Edinburgh: W. Oliphant, 1823.

Kerr, Anne Cecil. *Teresa Helena Higginson: Servant of God 'The Spouse of the Crucified' 1844-1905*. London: Sands & Co., 1927.

Kerr, Anne Cecil. *Teresa Helena Higginson, School Teacher and Mystic*. London: Sands & Co, 1928.

Kerr, Anne Cecil. *Teresa Helena Higginson, 1844-1906* [sic]. Dublin: Catholic Truth Society of Ireland, 1933.

Kerr, Anne Cecil. *Teresa Helena Higginson: de bruid van den gekruisigde 1844-1905*. The Hague / Antwerp: Pax, 1933.

Kerr, Anne Cecil. *Thérésa-Héléna Higginson, servante de Dieu épouse du crucifié; ou, La merveilleuse d'une institutrice libre anglaise*. Trad. Victor Bilée. Paris: Desclée de Brouwer, 1935.

Kerr, Anne Cecil. 'Letter to the editor'. *The Tablet*, 25 December 1937, 886.

Kershaw, Frederick W. *Teresa Helena Higginson: A Short Account of her Life and Letters*. London: Sands & Co., 1933.

Klein, Detmar. 'The Virgin with the Sword: Marian Apparitions, Religion and National Identity in Alsace in the 1870s'. *French History*, 21 (2007), 411-430.

Koch, Matthias. *Reise in Tirol in landschaftlicher und staatlicher Beziehung*. Mannheim: Bensheimer, 1852.

Kocherscheidt, Benjamin. *Deutsche Irrenärzte und Irrenseelsorger. Ein Beitrag zur Geschichte von Psychiatrie und Anstaltsseelsorge im 19. Jahrhundert*. Diss. Hamburg, 2010.

Kotulla, Andreas. *'Nach Lourdes!' Der französische Marienwallfahrtsort und die Katholiken im Deutschen Kaiserreich (1871-1914)*. Munich: Meidenaure, 2006.

Krieger, Leonard. 'The Idea of Authority in the West'. *The American Historical Review*, 82 (1977) 2, 249-270.

Kselman, Thomas A. *Miracles and Prophecies in Nineteenth-Century France*. New Brunswick / New Jersey: Rutgers University Press, 1983.

Kugelmann, Robert. *Psychology and Catholicism: Contested Boundaries*. Cambridge: Cambridge University Press, 2011.

Kugle, Scott. *Sufis and Saints' Bodies: Mysticism, Corporeality, and Sacred Power in Islam*. Chapel Hill: University of North Carolina Press, 2007.

Kutzer, Michael. 'Die therapeutischen Intentionen in der Irrenanstalt des 19. Jahrhunderts. Das Beispiel "Kloster Eberbach" (1815-1849)' in: Christina Vanja et al., eds. *Wissen und Irren. Psychiatriegeschichte aus zwei Jahrhunderten – Eberbach und Eichberg*. Kassel: Landeswohlfahrtsverband Hessen, 1999, 46-59.

Lachapelle, Sofie. 'Between Miracle and Sickness: Louise Lateau and the Experience of Stigmata and Ecstasy'. *Configurations*, 12 (2004), 77-105.

Laidley, W.S. 'Wizzard Clip'. *West Virginia Historical Magazine Quarterly*, January 1904. <https://archive.org/details/westvirginiahist04west>.

Lambing, Andrew Arnold. *A History of the Catholic Church in the Dioceses of Pittsburgh and Allegheny from its Establishment to the Present Time*. New York: Benziger Brothers, 1880. <http://digital.library.pitt.edu/cgi-bin/t/text/text-idx?idno=00aga8651m>.

Langlois, Claude. 'La photographie comme preuve entre médecine et religion'. *Histoire des sciences médicales*, 28 (1994) 4, 325-336.

Latour, Bruno. *We Have Never Been Modern*. Cambridge, Mass.: Harvard University Press, 1991.

Lederer, David. *Madness, Religion and the State in Early Modern Europe: A Bavarian Beacon*. Cambridge: Cambridge University Press, 2006.

Lentner, Ferdinand. *Sebastian Ruf. Irrenhaus-Kaplan zu Hall i. T. als Seelenforscher. Ein Beitrag zur Lehre von der Zurechnung im Strafrecht*. Innsbruck: Wagner, 1902.

Levitt, Peggy. 'Religion on the Move: Mapping Global Cultural Production and Consumption' in: Courtney Bender et al., eds. *Religion on the Edge: De-Centering and Re-Centering the Sociology of Religion*. New York: Oxford University Press, 2013, 159-176.

Lock, Margaret. 'Cultivating the Body: Anthropology and Epistemologies of Bodily Practice and Knowledge'. *Annual Review of Anthropology*, 22 (1993), 133 155.

Looney, Edward. 'Called to Evangelize: The Story of Adele Brise and the Mariophany that Changed her Life'. *Marian Studies*, 62 (2011), 119-138.

Lyon, F. Emory. Book review of J.S. Cammack, *Moral Problems of Mental Defect* in: *Journal of Criminal Law and Criminology*, 30 (March-April 1940), 976-978.

Maire, Laurence. *Les possédés de Morzine (1857-1873)*. Lyon: Presses Universitaires de Lyon, 1981.

Maistriaux, Fernand. *Que se passe-t-il à Beauraing?* Louvain: Rex, 1932.

Maistriaux, Fernand. *Les dernières apparitions de Beauraing*. Louvain: Rex, 1933.

Maître, Jacques. *Une inconnue célèbre: Madeleine Lebouc/Pauline Lair Lamotte (1863-1918)*. Paris: Anthropos, 1993.

Maître, Jacques. *Mystique et féminité. Essai de psychanalyse sociohistorique*. Paris: Cerf, 1997.

Maître, Jacques. 'De Bourneville à nos jours: interprétations psychiatriques de la mystique'. *L'Évolution psychiatrique*, 64 (1999), 765-778.

Marques, Tiago Pires. 'Mystique, politique et maladie mentale. Historicités croisées (France, c. 1830 - c. 1900)'. *Revue d'histoire des sciences humaines*, 23 (2010), 37-74.

Marques, Tiago Pires. 'De corpo e alma na margem: catolicismo, santidade e medicina no Norte de Portugal (c. 1900 - c. 1950)'. *Topoi* (Rio de Janeiro) [online], 13 (2012) 25, 147-167.

Marques, Tiago Pires. 'Uma frágil camada de Razão. A clínica das paixões religiosas em França e Portugal. C. 1830 - c. 1910' in: Tiago Pires Marques, ed. *Experiências à deriva. Paixões religiosas e psiquiatria na Europa (séculos XV a XXI)*. Lisbon: Cavalo de Ferro, 2013, 171-216.

Marques, Tiago Pires. 'Extraordinary Order: Fátima, Religious Affects and the Catholic Political Imagination in Portugal, c. 1910-1950'. *Portuguese Journal of Social Science*, 13 (2014) 3, 253-268.

Martindale, Cyril Charles. 'Letter to the Editor'. *The Tablet*, 22 January 1938, 119.

Mauchamp, Émile. *La Sorcellerie au Maroc. Œuvre Posthume*. Paris: Dorbon-Ainé, 1911.

Mauran, Dr. *La Société marocaine: Études sociales, impressions et souvenirs, avec une lettre-préface de M. Le Générale d'Amade, et une lettre de M. Guiot*. Paris: Paulin, 1910.

Mauriac, Emile and Henri Verdalle. *Étude médicale sur l'extatique de Fontet*. Paris: Germer Bailliere, 1875.

Mayer, Edward E. 'Hysteria in Children'. *Pennsylvania Medical Journal*, 2 (1899) 9, 480-481.

Mayeur, Jean-Marie. 'Mgr Dupanloup et Louis Veuillot devant les "prophéties contemporaines" en 1874'. *Revue d'histoire de la spiritualité*, 48 (1972), 193-204.

McGreevy, John T. 'Introduction: The American Catholic Century' in: R. Scott Appleby and Kathleen Sprows Cummings, eds. *Catholics in the American Century: Recasting Narratives of U.S. History*. Ithaca: Cornell University Press, 2012, 1-9.

McNabb, Vincent, ed. *Memorabilia: Gleanings from Father Wilberforce's Note Books*. London: Westminster Art & Book Company Ltd., 1910.

Micale, Mark S. *Approaching Hysteria: Disease and its Interpretations*. Princeton: Princeton University Press, 1995.

Minois, Georges. *L'Église et la science. Histoire d'un malentendu. De Galilée à Jean-Paul II*. Paris: Fayard, 1991.

Moisnard, Albert. 'Berguille. La voyante de Fontet'. *Le Gaulois*, 1 January 1875, 2-3.

Mollinger, Father S.G. *New York Times*, 1884-1892.

Monroe, John Warne. *Laboratories of Faith: Mesmerism, Spiritism, and Occultism in Modern France*. Ithaca: Cornell University Press, 2007.

Monydar, B. *Un doute sur la voyante de Fontet*. La Réole: E. Lecourt, 1874.

Morgan, David. *The Embodied Eye: Religious Visual Culture and the Social Life of Feeling*. Berkeley: University of California Press, 2012.

Moura, Elísio de. *Anorexia Mental*. Coimbra: Imprensa da Universidade de Coimbra, 2005 (1947).

Multon, Hilaire. 'Catholicisme intransigeant et culture prophétique: L'apport des archives du Saint-Office et de l'index'. *Revue historique*, 1 (2002) 621, 109-137.

Multon, Hilaire. 'Prophétesses et prophéties dans la seconde moitié du pontificat de Pie IX (1859-78). Entre défense du pouvoir temporel et apocalypse hétérodoxe'. *Dimensioni e problemi della ricera storica*, 1 (2003), 131-159.

Multon, Hilaire. 'Faire de la politique du miracle. L'abbé Jean-Marie Curique (diocèse de Metz, 1827-1892), restaurateur de sites religieux et compilateur de prophéties'. *Chrétiens et sociétés*, 12 (2005), 59-70.

Nicaise-Vermer, P. *Apparitions de la Vierge à Beauraing. Accusés, levez-vous!* Brussels: Lesigne, 1933.

Niedermeyer, Albert. *Handbuch der speziellen Pastoralmedizin. 5: Seelenleiden und Seelenheilung (Psychopathologie und Psychotherapie)*. Vienna: Herder, 1952.

Nolte, Karen and Fangerau, Heiner. 'Einleitung: "Moderne" Anstaltspsychiatrie im 19. und 20. Jahrhundert – Legitimation und Kritik' in: Heiner Fangerau and Karen Nolte, eds. *"Moderne" Anstaltspsychiatrie im 19. und 20. Jahrhundert – Legitimation und Kritik*. Stuttgart: Franz Steiner Verlag, 2006, 7-21.

Nordqvist, Christian. 'What are symptoms? What are signs?'. *Medical News Today*. MediLexicon, Intl., 8 Sept. 2014. <http://www.medicalnewstoday.com/articles/161858.php> [10 October 2014].

Nys, Liesbet et al., eds. *De zieke natie. Over de medicalisering van de samenleving 1860-1914*. Groningen: Historische Uitgeverij, 2002.

Orsi, Robert. *Between Heaven and Earth: The Religious Worlds People Make and the Scholars Who Study Them*. Princeton: Princeton University Press, 2005.

Orsi, Robert. 'U.S. Catholics between Memory and Modernity: How Catholics are American' in: R. Scott Appleby and Kathleen Sprows Cummings, eds, *Catholics in the American Century: Recasting Narratives of U.S. History*. Ithaca: Cornell University Press, 2012, 11-42.

Ossa-Richardson, Anthony. 'Possession or Insanity? Two Views from the Victorian Lunatic Asylum'. *Journal of the History of Ideas*, 74 (2013) 4, 553-575.

O'Sullivan, Adalbert M. *Teresa Higginson, the Servant of God, School Teacher*. London: Sands & Co., 1924.

Park, Karen E. 'The Negotiation of Authority at a Frontier Marian Apparition Site: Adele Brise and Our Lady of Good Help'. *American Catholic Studies*, 123 (2012) 3, 1-26.

Paul, Harry. *From Knowledge to Power: The Rise of the Science Empire in France, 1860-1939*. Cambridge: Cambridge University Press, 1985.

Péladan, Adrien. *Ma retraite du châtiment, suivie des dernières prédictions de la voyante de Fontet*. Nîmes: Chez les librairies, 1874.

Péladan, Adrien. *(Suite à Dernier mot des Prophéties) Évènements miraculeux de Fontet, de Blain et de Marpingen. Prophéties authentiques des voyantes contemporaines Berguille et Marie-Julie*. Nîmes: Chez l'auteur, 1878.

Péladan, Adrien. *Dernier mot des prophéties ou l'avenir prochain dévoilé par plusieurs centaines de textes authentiques, dont beaucoup sont peu connus ou inédits et de date récente*. Nîmes: Chez l'auteur, 1881.

Pise, Charles Constantine. *Father Rowland: A North American Tale*. Baltimore: Fielding Lucas, Jr., 1829.

Pitts, Ann and Dolores, Mary. *Teresa Helena Higginson: Servant of God*. Neston: Mrs G.M. Moreton, 17 Sidney Road, 1986.

Pompey, Heinrich. *Die Bedeutung der Medizin für die kirchliche Seelsorge im Selbstverständnis der sogenannten Pastoralmedizin. Eine bibliographische-historische Untersuchung*. Freiburg/Vienna: Herder, 1968.

Porter, Roy. 'Religion and Medicine' in: William F. Bynum and Roy Porter, eds. *Companion Encyclopaedia of the History of Medicine*. London: Routledge, 1993, 1449-1469.

Portets, V. de. *Lettres sur la voyante de Fontet. Première série*. Agen: André Roche, 1874.

Portets, V. de. *Lettres sur la voyante de Fontet. Deuxième série*. Agen: André Roche, 1874.

Portets, V. de. *La résurrection de Berguille, suite aux Lettres sur la voyante de Fontet, avec le récit de l'éclatante guérison du 2 août 1875*. Lyon: H. Pélagaud et Roblot, 1875.

Priesching, Nicole, ed. *Unter der Geisel Gottes. Das Leiden der stigmatisierten Maria von Mörl (1812-1868) im Urteil ihres Beichtvaters*. Brixen: Weger, 2007.

Priesching, Nicole. 'Mystikerinnen des 19. Jahrhunderts - ein neuer Typus?' in: Waltraud Pulz, ed. *Zwischen Himmel und Erde. Körperliche Zeichen der Heiligkeit*. Stuttgart: Franz Steiner Verlag, 2012, 79-97.

Pulz, Waltraud. 'Krank versus gesund? Von heilsamer Krankheit und körperlichen Zeichen der Heiligkeit' in: Michael Simon, ed. *Auf der Suche nach Heil und Heilung. Religiöse Aspekte der medikalen Alltagskultur*. Dresden: Thelem, 2011, 73-85.

Pulz, Waltraud. 'Vorbemerkung' in: Waltraud Pulz, ed. *Zwischen Himmel und Erde. Körperliche Zeichen der Heiligkeit*. Stuttgart: Franz Steiner Verlag, 2012, 7-13.

Rahnema, Ali. *An Islamic Utopian: A Political Biography of Ali Shariati*. London: I. B. Tauris, 2014.

Rainford, Margaret M. 'Letter to the Editor'. *Catholic Herald*, 19 June 2009, 13.

Regnard, Paul and Bourneville, Désiré Magloire. *Iconographie photographique de la Salpêtrière (service de M. Charcot)*. Paris: Bureaux du 'Progrès médical', 1876-1880, 3 vols.

Reil, Johann Christian. *Rhapsodieen* über *die Anwendung der psychischen Kurmethode auf Geisteszerrüttungen*. Halle: Curtsche Buchhandlung, 1803.

La résurrection de la France et le châtiment de la Prusse prédits par Marie en Alsace & à Fontet. Paris: Aldophe Josse, 1874.

Richer, Paul. *Études cliniques sur l'hystéro-épilepsie ou grade hystérie*. Paris: Delahaye et Lecrosnier, 1885.
Ricken, David. 'Decree on the Authenticity of the Apparitions of 1858 at the Shrine of Our Lady of Good Help'. 2010. <shrineofourladyofgood-help.com>.
Rivet, Daniel. *Lyautey et l'institution du protectorat français au Maroc, 1912-1925*. Paris: L'Harmattan, 1996, 3 vols.
Robertson, Roland. 'Glocalization: Time-Space and Homogeneity-Heterogeneity' in: Mike Featherstone, Scott Lash and Roland Robertson, eds. *Global Modernities*. London: Sage Publications, 1995, 25-44.
Rose, Janet. *The Woman who Claimed to be Christ: The Millennial Belief of Mary Ann Girling and her Disciples, 1860-1886*. DPhil. diss. Oxford, 2008.
Ruf, Sebastian. 'Gymnastische Uebung. Erziehung zur Arbeit'. *Volks- und Schützenzeitung für Tirol und Vorarlberg*, 4 February 1853.

Sarasin, Philipp. 'Was ist Wissensgeschichte?' *Internationales Archiv für Sozialgeschichte der deutschen Literatur*, 36 (2011), 159-172.
Saurer, Edith. 'Frauen und Priester. Beichtgespräche im frühen 19. Jahrhundert' in: Richard van Dülmen, ed. *Arbeit, Frömmigkeit und Eigensinn. Studien zur historischen Kulturforschung*, vol. 2. Frankfurt am Main: Fischer Taschenbuch, 1990, 141-170.
Scheer, Monique. 'Verspielte Frömmigkeit: Somatische Interaktionen beim Marienerscheinungskult von Heroldsbach-Thurn 1949/50'. *Historische Anthropologie*, 17 (2009) 3, 386-405.
Scheer, Monique. 'Das Medium hat ein Geschlecht' in: Hubert Wolf, ed. *'Wahre' und 'falsche' Heiligkeit. Mystik, Macht und Geschlechterrollen im Katholizismus des 19. Jahrhunderts*. Oldenburg, 2013, 169-192.
Scheer, Monique. 'What She Looks Like: On the Recognition and Iconization of the Virgin Mary at Apparition Sites in the Twentieth Century'. *Material Religion. The Journal of Objects, Art and Belief*, 9 (2013) 4, 442-467.
Schloesser, Steve. *Jazz Age Catholicism: Mystic Modernism in Postwar Paris, 1919-1933*. Toronto: University of Toronto Press, 2005.
Schneider, Bernhard. 'Marienerscheinungen im 19. Jahrhundert' in: Hubert Wolf, ed. *'Wahre' und 'falsche' Heiligkeit. Mystik, Macht und Geschlechterrollen im Katholizismus des 19. Jahrhunderts*. Oldenburg, 2013, 87-110.
Schön, Bruno. *Mittheilungen aus dem Leben Geistesgestörter*. Pest / Vienna / Leipzig: Verlag C.A. Hartleben, 1859.
Schultz, Nancy Lusignan. *Mrs. Mattingly's Miracle: The Prince, the Widow, and the Cure that Shocked Washington City*. New Haven: Yale University Press, 2011.
Shrine of Our Lady of Good Help. <www.shrineofourladyofgoodhelp.com>.
La semaine religieuse du diocèse de Rouen. Rouen, 25 December 1875.
Spadola, Emilio. 'The Scandal of Ecstasy: Communication, Sufi Rites, and Social Reform in 1930s Morocco'. *Contemporary Islam*, 2 (2008) 2, 119-138.
Steub, Ludwig. *Sängerkrieg in Tirol. Erinnerungen aus den Jahren 1842-1844*. Stuttgart: Adolf Bonz & Comp., 1882.
Stolberg, Michael. '"Volksfromme" Heilpraktiken und medikale Alltagskultur im Bayern des 19. Jahrhunderts' in: Michael Simon, ed. *Auf der Suche nach Heil und Heilung. Religiöse Aspekte der medikalen Alltagskultur*. Dresden, 2011, 155-173.
Stolz, Josef. 'Zur fortschreitenden Parese'. *Allgemeine Zeitschrift für Psychiatrie*, 8 (1851), 517-559.
Stolz, Josef. 'Aerztlicher Bericht der k. k. Irren-Anstalt zu Hall in Tyrol über das Militärjahr 1860'. *Allgemeine Zeitschrift für Psychiatrie*, 18 (1861), 581-595.
Summers, Montague. *The Physical Phenomena of Mysticism with Especial Reference to the Stigmata, Divine and Diabolic*. London: Rider and Company, 1950.
Szabo, Jason. 'Seeing is Believing? The Form and Substance of French Medical Debates over Lourdes'. *Bulletin of the History of Medicine*, 76 (2002), 199-230.

'A Teacher Saint'. *The Catholic Herald*, 27 November 1936, 14.
'Teacher's Friend'. Letter to the Editor. *The Tablet*, 11 December 1937, 803.
Tenbus, Eic. *English Catholics and the Education of the Poor, 1847-1902*. London: Pickering and Chatto, 2010.
Terças, José Alves. 'A martirizada do Calvário'. *Vida de Cristo, a Paixão Dolorosa*, 5 (Lisbon, 1941) 10.
Thurston, Herbert. 'Hagiography: Past and Present'. *The Tablet*, 20 November 1937, 683-684.
Thurston, Herbert. 'Teresa Higginson'. *The Tablet*, 11 December 1937, 803.

Thurston, Herbert. 'Beatification: An Historical Account of the Processes of Beatification and Canonization'. *The Tablet*, 15 January 1938, 72-73.
Thurston, Herbert. 'Letter to the Editor'. *The Tablet*, 29 January 1938, 151.
Thurston, Herbert. *The Physical Phenomena of Mysticism*. Ed. J.H. Crehan. London: Burns and Oates, 1952.
Torgal, Luís Filipe. *O Sol bailou ao Meio-Dia: A Criação de Fátima*. Lisbon: Tinta da China, 2011.
Trillat, Emile. 'Introduction' in: Jean-Martin Charcot. *L'hystérie*. Paris: L'Harmattan, 1998.
Tschallener, Johann. *Beschreibung der k. k. Provinzial-Irren-Heilanstalt zu Hall in Tirol mit Rücksicht auf die Statuten der Anstalt, auf die therapeutischen und psychologischen Grundsätze der Behandlung der Geisteskranken und auf ihre achtjährigen Resultate*. Innsbruck: Wagner, 1842.
Tunhas, Paulo. 'Três tipos de crenças' in: Fernando Gil, Pierre Livet and João Pina Cabral, eds. *O processo da crença*. Lisbon: Gradiva, 2004, 119-134.

Van Acker, K. 'Beauraing'. *Vlaamsch Geneeskundig Tijdschrift*, 14 (1933) 23, 445-454.
Van Hoestenberghe, L.; Royer, E. and Deschamps, A. 'Récit et étude d'une guérison subite de fracture'. *Revue des questions scientifiques*, October 1899, 516-560.
Vanja, Christina. 'Madhouses, Children's Wards, and Clinics: The Development of Insane Asylums in Germany' in: Norbert Finzsch and Robert Jütte, eds. *Institutions of Confinement. Hospitals, Asylums, and Prisons in Western Europe and North America, 1500-1950*. Washington, D.C.: Cambridge University Press, 1996, 117-132.
Vanja, Christina. 'Die Irrenanstalt muss in einer anmutigen Gegend liegen. Über die Gründung der Herzoglich Nassauischen Heil- und Pflegeanstalt Eichberg' in: Christina Vanja et al., eds. *Wissen und Irren. Psychiatriegeschichte aus zwei Jahrhunderten – Eberbach und Eichberg*. Kassel: Landeswohlfahrtsverband Hessen, 1999, 11-35.
Vanja, Christina. 'Das Irrenhaus als Totale Institution? Erving Goffmans Modell aus psychiatriehistorischer Perspektive' in: Martin Scheutz, ed. *Totale Institutionen*. Wiener Zeitschrift zur Geschichte der Neuzeit, 8, 1. Innsbruck: Studienverlag, 2008, 120-129.
Velle, Karel. 'Het verenigingsleven van de Belgische geneesheer (19de en begin 20ste eeuw), een bijdrage tot de geschiedenis van het artsenberoep'. *Annales de la Société belge d'histoire des hôpitaux et de la santé publique*, 26-27 (1988-1989), 47-118.
Velle, Karel. 'De geneeskunde en de R.K. Kerk (1830-1940): een moeilijke verhouding?'. *Trajecta*, 4 (1995) 1, 1-21.
Veloso, Agostinho. 'A Mística e a Medicina'. *Brotéria*, January 1942.
Veloso, Agostinho. 'Mística e jornalismo'. *Brotéria*, January 1947, 5-20.
'A Vice-Postulator'. Letter to the Editor. *The Tablet*, 19 February 1938, 247.
'La voyante de Fontet'. *Annales catholiques: Revue religieuse hebdomadaire de la France et de l'Église*, 22 January 1975, 217-218.

Walshe, Francis M.R. 'Teresa Higginson'. *The Tablet*, 8 May 1937, 665-666.
Walshe, Francis M.R. 'Letter to the Editor'. *The Tablet*, 29 January 1938, 150.
Walshe, Francis M.R. 'Letter to the Editor'. *The Tablet*, 26 February 1938, 277-278.
Waugh, Evelyn. 'Letter to the Editor'. *The Tablet*, 11 December 1937, 803.
Weiß, Otto. 'Seherinnen und Stigmatisierte' in: Irmtraud Götz von Olenhusen, ed. *Wunderbare Erscheinungen. Frauen und katholische Frömmigkeit im 19. und 20. Jahrhundert*. Paderborn: Schöningh, 1995, 51-82.
Weiß, Otto. *Weisungen aus dem Jenseits? Der Einfluss mystizistischer Phänomene auf Ordens- und Kirchenleitungen im 19. Jahrhundert*. Regensburg: Pustet, 2011.
Weiß, Otto. 'Stigmata' in: Hubert Wolf, ed. *'Wahre' und 'falsche' Heiligkeit. Mystik, Macht und Geschlechterrollen im Katholizismus des 19. Jahrhunderts*. Oldenburg: Oldenbourg Verlag, 2013, 111-125.
Westerink, Herman. 'Demonic Possession and the Historical Construction of Melancholy and Hysteria'. *History of Psychiatry*, 25 (2014) 3, 335-349.
Whittington-Egan, Richard. *The Devil in Bootle: The Life and Afterlife of Teresa Higginson*. Liverpool: The Bluecoat Press, 2010.
Worlock, Derek. 'Requiem address for Douglas Woodruff'. *The Tablet*, 18 March 1978, 36-38.

Ziemann, Benjamin. 'Säkularisierung, Konfessionalisierung, Organisationsbildung. Dimensionen der Sozialgeschichte der Religion im langen 19. Jahrhundert'. *Archiv für Sozialgeschichte*, 47 (2007), 485-508.

Zimdars-Swartz, Sandra L. *Encountering Mary: From La Salette to Medjugorje*. Princeton, N.J.: Princeton University Press, 1991.

Zumholz, Maria Anna. 'Die Resistenz des katholischen Milieus: Seherinnen und Stigmatisierte in der ersten Hälfte des 20. Jahrhunderts' in: Irmtraud Götz von Olenhusen, ed. *Wunderbare Erscheinungen. Frauen und katholische Frömmigkeit im 19. und 20. Jahrhundert*. Paderborn: Schöningh, 1995, 221-251.

Zumholz, Maria Anna. *Volksfrömmigkeit und katholisches Milieu. Marienerscheinungen in Heede 1937-1949*. Cloppenburg: Runge, 2004.

INDEX OF NAMES

CONTRIBUTORS

Ellen J. Amster is the Jason A. Hannah Chair in the History of Medicine at McMaster University in Ontario, Canada, and an associate professor in the Department of Clinical Epidemiology and Biostatistics and the Department of History. Her research touches upon non-Western health and healing systems, traditional midwifery, phenomenology of the body, the modern history of public health, Islamic science, French and Islamic medical histories, and the physical geographies of Sufism. (E.g. *Medicine and the Saints: Science, Islam and the Colonial Encounter in Morocco, 1877-1956*. Austin: University of Texas Press, 2013). Her current research projects include a study of Islamic sainthood, a translation from Arabic to English of a nineteenth-century Moroccan hagiographical compendium by Muhammad ibn Ja'far al-Kattani, and shrine architecture in the city of Fez.

Henk de Smaele is associate professor of History at the University of Antwerp, where he is affiliated to Power in History: Centre for Political History. He is also Chair of the Antwerp Research Institute for the Arts (ARIA). His research interests include the modern history of gender and sexuality, as well as the relationships between the Middle East and Europe in the nineteenth and twentieth centuries. He recently co-edited (with Edhem Eldem and Houssine Alloul) *To Kill a Sultan: A Transnational History of the Attempt on Abdülhamid II (1905)* (Palgrave Macmillan, 2017).

Nicole Edelman is honorary senior lecturer/associate professor (Maîtresse de conferences) of Contemporary History (Paris Ouest Nanterre, HAR). Her research focuses on fields often forgotten or side-lined by mainstream historians and by the political, scientific and religious establishment. She has published on different phenomena, such as hypnosis, magnetic somnambulism, trances, and other states of altered consciousness and other cultural, intellectual and religious phenomena. In the recent years, her work has shifted toward the history of psychiatry, psychology and psychoanalysis, mainly in the nineteenth century.

Maria Heidegger is holding the Erika-Cremer Post-Doctoral Fellowship at the Department of History and European Ethnology at the University of Innsbruck. Her research interests include the history of psychiatry, the social history of medicine and religion, as well as the history of gender relations. Latest publications are 'Landscapes of Psychiatry in the Tyrol in the Nineteenth Century with a Comparative View of Louisiana' in: C. Antenhofer et al. (eds.), *Cities as Multiple Landscapes: Investigating the Sister Cities Innsbruck and New Orleans* (Frankfurt/New York: Campus, 2016, 471-494), and '"Fromme" Lektüre, "scharfe" Predigt: Zur Problematisierung religiöser Praktiken in Krankenakten der k. k. Provinzial-Irrenanstalt Hall in Tirol, 1830-1850', in: *Virus. Beiträge zur Sozialgeschichte der Medizin*, 15 (2016), 127-150.

Mary Heimann is professor of Modern History at Cardiff University in Wales. She is the author of *Catholic Devotion in Victorian England* (Oxford: Oxford University Press, 1995); 'Christianity in Western Europe from the Enlightenment to the Present Day' in: Adrian Hastings, ed., *A World History of Christianity* (London: Cassell, 1999, 458-507) and *Czechoslovakia: The State that Failed* (New Haven: Yale University Press, 2009). Her research interests include English Catholic spirituality, modern mysticism and Catholic-Communist relations in Cold War Czechoslovakia, Hungary and Poland.

Paula Kane is John and Lucine O'Brien Marous Chair of Catholic Studies at the University of Pittsburgh. She teaches courses on American religious history, religion and film, religion and globalization, popular religion and Catholic Studies. Her most recent book, *Sister Thorn and Catholic Mysticism in Modern America* (Chapel Hill: University of North Carolina Press, 2013), studies an alleged stigmatic nun in New York in the 1920s.

Sofie Lachapelle is associate professor of History at the University of Guelph. She is the author of *Conjuring Science: A History of Scientific Entertainment and Stage Magic in Modern France* (New York: Palgrave MacMillan, 2015) and *Investigating the Supernatural: From Spiritism and Occultism to Psychical Research and Metapsychics in France, 1853-1931* (Baltimore: Johns Hopkins University Press, 2011). She is presently working on a project dealing with the relationship of opera, vocal pedagogy, and medicine in late-nineteenth-century France.

Tiago Pires Marques is a researcher at the Center for Social Studies (University of Coimbra). He is the author of *Crime and the Fascist State. 1950-1940* (Routledge, 2015) and currently focuses on medical and religious forms of objectivizing and communicating psychic suffering. His recent publications include: *Michel de Certeau et l'anthropologie historique de la modernité* (issue of the *Revue d'histoire des sciences humaines*, 23 (2010) 2; co-ordinator) and *Experiências à deriva. Paixões religiosas e psiquiatria na Europa (séculos XV a XXI)* (Lisbon: Cavalo de Ferro, 2013).

Tine Van Osselaer is research professor in the history of spirituality, devotion and mysticism at the Ruusbroec Institute of the University of Antwerp. She has published on gender and religion (*The Pious Sex: Catholic Constructions of Masculinity and Femininity in Belgium, c. 1800-1940.* Leuven: Leuven University Press, 2013); religion and the family, and on corporeality and emotions. Currently, she is the principal investigator of STIGMATICS: 'Between saints and celebrities. The devotion and promotion of stigmatics in Europe, c. 1800-1950', a project sponsored by the European Research Council (Starting Grant).

Kaat Wils is professor in Contemporary Cultural History at the University of Leuven, where she leads the Research Group Cultural History since 1750. Her research interests are modern intellectual history, history of the humanities and the biomedical sciences, gender history and history education. She recently coedited *Scientists' Expertise as Performance: Between State and Society, 1860-1960* (London: Pickering & Chatto, 2015) and *Bodies Beyond Borders. Moving Anatomies 1750-1950* (Leuven: Leuven University Press, 2017).

COLOPHON

FINAL EDITING
Luc Vints

COPY EDITING
Lieve Claes

LAY-OUT
Alexis Vermeylen

KADOC
Documentation and Research Centre for Religion, Culture and Society
Vlamingenstraat 39
B - 3000 Leuven
www.kadoc.kuleuven.be

Leuven University Press
Minderbroedersstraat 4
B - 3000 Leuven
www.lup.be